STAYING
ALIVE

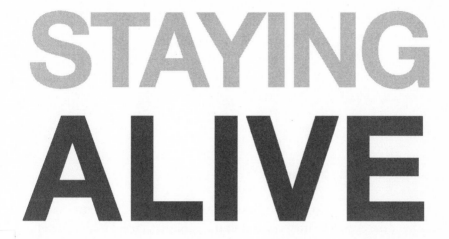

STAYING ALIVE

The Signs That You Have to See a Doctor Right Now
(and the Ways to Avoid Having to See One Again)

MATTHEW HAHN, MD

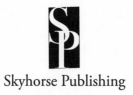

Skyhorse Publishing

Skyhorse Publishing books may be purchased in bulk at special discounts for sales promotion, corporate gifts, fund-raising, or educational purposes. Special editions can also be created to specifications. For details, contact the Special Sales Department, Skyhorse Publishing, 307 West 36th Street, 11th Floor, New York, NY 10018 or info@skyhorsepublishing.com.

Skyhorse® and Skyhorse Publishing® are registered trademarks of Skyhorse Publishing, Inc.®, a Delaware corporation.

Visit our website at www.skyhorsepublishing.com.
10 9 8 7 6 5 4 3 2 1

Library of Congress Cataloging-in-Publication Data is available on file.

Cover design by Rain Saukas
Cover photo: iStockphoto

Print ISBN: 978-1-5107-1395-6
Ebook ISBN: 978-1-5107-1396-3

Printed in the United States of America

CONTENTS

INTRODUCTION

This may be the most important medical book you will ever read. I hope it might also be one of the most interesting.

My ultimate hope for this book is that it will save lives—that it will help people to beat the odds. The current odds when it comes to your health are that you will die from the effects of one of the following common but often preventable conditions—heart disease, stroke, diabetes, or cancer. The odds also predict that one in every three children born in America will develop diabetes during their lifetime, that two-thirds of American adults will be overweight, and that one-half of those people will be overweight to the point of being obese.

The practice of medicine, as I have come to understand it, is an attempt to increase the odds that a patient will live a long, healthy life. That's what this book is about.

It is no secret, though, that health care in America is in disarray. My concern is that something very important gets lost in the uproar of arguing the causes and possible solutions to this very great mess.

What can get lost is that modern health care offers many true miracles—if you can take advantage of them. And despite the difficulties in accessing health care faced by so many in America today, the most important of these miracles are readily available and affordable for just about everyone.

Modern health care is also criticized for being too focused on treating illness, and not enough on promoting health and wellness. The point is well taken.

The best approach balances the two—successfully evaluating and treating illnesses when they arise, while at the same time making every effort to keep patients well. In other words, to beat the odds, we must treat the treatable and prevent the preventable!

Staying Alive: The Signs That You Have to See a Doctor Right Now (and the Ways to Avoid Having to See One Again) is your guide to beating the odds when it comes to your health. If you really want to do so, you must do all three of the following:

1. Most important—by a very long shot—we optimize our chances of being healthy and staying well by eating right, by exercising regularly, by not smoking, and by avoiding excessive alcohol use.
2. We must take advantage of the miracles available today through modern preventive medical care.

Despite our best efforts, and despite even the best of preventive care, the reality is that illness and injuries still occur. Therefore, we must also:

3. Get medical care when it is necessary, in the hope that treatable conditions are identified early enough that they can still be treated.

The problem is:

1. Too many people delay until it is too late when signs of serious (but treatable) illness first appear.
2. Many people fail to receive—or worse, they refuse—many of the most important preventive treatments available because they do not understand the revolutionary developments that have taken place in preventive medical care.
3. The great majority of people don't eat well or exercise regularly.

Staying Alive: The Signs That You Have to See a Doctor Right Now (and the Ways to Avoid Having to See One Again) is the ultimate modern health-care survival guide because it uniquely addresses each of these issues. It is a three-part guide to optimal health and wellness and to surviving illness for the modern patient.

1. **Sixty-Two Medical Complaints That Should Never Be Ignored.** As part of their medical education, doctors are taught that there are certain classic symptoms that, until proven otherwise, are the first signs of a serious medical condition that requires urgent or even emergency treatment. What I see all too often is that when such symptoms develop, patients delay care, usually because they do not understand the significance of their circumstances, and preventable tragedy ensues.

   The intent of this section is *to teach you those important signs and symptoms so that you know when you absolutely need to see a doctor and how quickly you need to get there.*

2. **The Miracles of Twenty-First-Century Medicine: Taking Advantage of Modern Preventive Medical Care.** A revolution has taken place in the medical sciences. We can now prevent and/or successfully treat many of the most serious common medical conditions that just a short time ago would make us ill and even kill us. The problem is that many people harbor negative attitudes regarding modern medical care, and therefore do not receive safe, truly lifesaving, and readily available treatments. In this important section, you will learn about the true miracle that is modern preventive medical care.

3. **The *Be Healthy! Workbook*: Optimizing Eating and Exercise to Promote Wellness and Prevent Disease.** The true secret to health and wellness is healthy eating and regular exercise. And yet, so few of us do this. There is no pill, no herb, no supplement, nor any magic bullet that has been shown to reliably lower our risks of significant illness in any comparable way. The *Be Healthy! Workbook* provides a simple, systematic method to develop and maintain healthy eating and exercise habits. Developed through years of working directly with patients, the

key to the approach described in the *Be Healthy! Workbook* is simplicity. The potential payoff for your health is immense.

Combining all three—getting care when necessary; taking advantage of the full benefits of modern preventive care; and, most importantly, eating well and exercising, every person can maximize the odds that they will live a long, healthy, and happy life. *Staying Alive* was written specifically to help you do just that.

This true story says it all:

The patient was an early middle-aged man, married with children. He hadn't been to the doctor in years. He had been feeling well until he experienced the sudden onset of severe, crushing pain in his chest. His wife transported him to our office.

The patient was so uncomfortable that he could not get out of his truck. So my nurse, Tonya, and I made a truck call!

He was sitting in the passenger seat, holding himself rigidly to combat the intense pain. He was pale and sweating. The pain in his chest radiated up to his jaw and made breathing uncomfortable.

Practicing in a small town, miles from the nearest large hospital, my staff and I are used to seeing patients when they develop chest pain. This was the most ill-appearing patient with chest pain we had ever seen. He had the classic appearance of a man having a heart attack. He looked like he might be dying.

Per our protocol, we contacted emergency medical services, gave him nitroglycerin, and had him chew an aspirin.

His pulse was weak and fast. I considered asking Tonya to get our defibrillator, just in case he went into cardiac arrest.

The ambulance arrived quickly. The patient was transported to the hospital 25 miles away. I spoke to the ER triage nurse to review the details of the case.

That evening, on the way home, I contacted the ER and spoke to the physician who was seeing our patient. The ER physician said that the patient was looking quite a bit more comfortable than when we had seen him at our office. I explained how badly he had looked previously and asked to be called when the results of the workup were available.

What is really interesting is that I don't always make a call like that.

I received a call back from the ER physician at about 9:00 p.m. A standard workup had not revealed any sign of a heart attack. The patient was feeling much better and really wanted to leave. The ER physician was wondering if that would be OK, and if we could follow up with the patient to complete the workup later with a stress test.

I had a bad feeling, though, and I urged them to keep him longer. Much to her credit, the ER physician heard something in what I was saying. Together with the patient's wife, she persuaded the patient to stay.

He was admitted for further observation. Fortunately, the hospitalist who picked up the case viewed the patient's condition from a fresh perspective and ordered a CAT scan of his chest.

This was not a heart attack. It was worse. The patient had an aortic dissection, one of the most feared diagnoses we can make. An aortic dissection is a tearing of the wall of the aorta, the largest blood vessel in the body, which comes directly from the heart. A huge percentage of people with an aortic dissection die immediately, before receiving care. The cause of an aortic dissection is usually untreated high blood pressure, which puts undue stress on the walls of the body's blood vessels.

Surgery—very complicated and risky surgery—was performed. Our patient lived. He has recovered very well.

This is a miracle. It is a true miracle of our times. It is a miracle that very nearly did not happen.

Most people know chest pain might be a sign of a heart attack. And yet, many people ignore this important symptom. In this case, had our patient waited to come in when he developed chest pain, he almost surely would have died. Had he left the ER before the diagnosis had been made, he would have died. Had he not received an amazing array of diagnostic tests and treatments, he would have died. He is alive, and we expect him to make a full recovery.

Now we have to keep him well, so he doesn't end up right back where he started. His blood pressure is now being monitored regularly and treated with medication that will significantly lower the odds that another dissection will occur. Most importantly, he is eating better and exercising regularly, which will do more than anything to lower his risks of a recurrence.

In this one story, we see it all—*Staying Alive*. Miracles can happen when we:

1. Get medical care when it is needed.
2. Receive the full benefits of preventive medical care.
3. Eat healthy and exercise.

PART 1

Sixty-Two Medical Complaints That Should Never Be Ignored

Chapter 1

Introduction

As part of their medical education, doctors are taught about classic symptoms that must be recognized because they may be the first sign of an urgent or even emergency medical condition. When such circumstances arise, delaying medical care risks life and limb. For instance:

- A patient who says she has "the worst headache of my life" is presumed to have a bleed in the brain (subarachnoid hemorrhage) until proven otherwise.
- Vaginal bleeding that occurs in a woman who has already gone through menopause is a sign of uterine cancer until proven otherwise.
- A one-sided headache accompanied by tenderness of the scalp in a person over the age of 50 may be a sign of "giant cell arteritis," a condition that can cause blindness if not diagnosed and treated in time.
- Low back pain that is accompanied by numbness of the groin and buttocks and difficulty controlling the bowels or bladder may be an indication of a condition known as the "cauda equina syndrome," which, if not treated very quickly, can result in permanent paralysis.

Knowing when to seek medical care is an extraordinarily important skill that is underappreciated and underaddressed by the multitude of self-help medical books available.

The purpose of this section is *to teach you those important signs and symptoms*—to help you stay alive! I want to alert people who may have little or no medical training to key medical symptoms that should never be ignored and give guidance regarding how quickly medical care is needed when those symptoms appear.

This is not a guide to medical self-diagnosis or self-care. Forgive me, but what I have observed through years of patient care is that patients very rarely make good self-diagnosticians (or family diagnosticians). Most people lack the objectivity and experience necessary to make an appropriate diagnosis, especially when they are attempting to self-diagnose.

This is not an emergency medical or first aid guide. Many obvious emergencies, such as broken bones and other forms of trauma, like cuts and bumps, are not discussed. I assume that if there is blood spurting or a bone sticking out, you will know to get yourself to the emergency room. The situations included in this section may not be quite as obvious or may require judgment in deciding when to seek medical care.

The goal here is simpler and I think more important and more achievable: to teach you when and how quickly you need to seek medical care. That is what is different about the material in *Sixty-Two Medical Complaints That Should Never Be Ignored.* And the information is easily digestible so that every person can learn this most valuable and potentially lifesaving skill in a short amount of time.

In addition, I would like to teach people skills that will enable them to more effectively interact and communicate with their health-care team (which could also save your life) and to prepare patients to deal with an increasingly crazed, confusing, and often confounding American health-care system.

Sixty-Two Medical Complaints That Should Never Be Ignored is divided into two sections:

1. *When to See the Doctor: The Cardinal Signs and Symptoms of Disease.* After an introductory section entitled "General Rules of Thumb," complaints are organized by body part, arranged

roughly from head to toe. There is also a section that focuses specifically on "Newborns, Babies, and Infants."

Each complaint includes a "Threat Level" to make the seriousness of each situation as clear as possible:

- LOW Threat Level: requires medical attention in one to four weeks.
- MEDIUM Threat Level: should receive medical attention within one week.
- HIGH Threat Level: should receive same-day medical attention.
- VERY HIGH Threat Level: an urgent situation that requires medical attention within one to six hours.
- HIGHEST Threat Level: a true emergency that requires immediate medical attention.

The following disclaimer applies, however. No matter the Threat Level listed, the more severe a symptom, the more quickly medical attention may be necessary. In addition, any symptom accompanied by signs of severe illness or distress requires immediate attention. When in doubt, call the doctor.

2. *Organizing Your Medical Information.* Understanding how best to maintain your past medical information and to discuss your medical problems with your medical team may save your life. This section is a guide to organizing your past medical information (the same way that doctors do) and to communicating the details of your medical complaints when you see the doctor.

The material in this section is intentionally brief so that with just a quick read, you will have the knowledge you need to be a smarter and safer (if not better-looking) patient. It is organized in a logical fashion so that it can also be used, in cases of an important, urgent, or even emergency situation, as a quick reference guide to inform readers what they need to do.

I hope you will also indulge me. I think it will be worth your while. I have tried to make the material interesting and, when possible, even entertaining. The study of medicine is serious but all too often technical and boring as well. At the end of each section, I have included illustrative and amusing anecdotes from my real-life practice in the hopes that an entertaining and interesting read might be more engaging. It is never my intent to make fun of patients, but it is often my intent to have fun with patients. If an incident about which I was writing took place recently, and/or I thought it was remotely possible that the patient could be identified from the story's details, I obtained permission from the patient to write the story. You can also assume that if I used a patient's name, I had permission to do so. The stories are true to the best of my recollection. Rarely, I changed minor details to protect the anonymity of the subject.

Why People Avoid Seeking Medical Care

For a variety of reasons, some of which make sense and many of which do not, people avoid going to the doctor when they need to go. What I see too often is people who wait too long when time is (or was) of the essence. Some of the reasons people avoid going to the doctor:

- **Didn't know any better.** This is common (and understandable). I hope that it's less common after this book comes out.
- **Thought they knew better.** It's just so easy to get an appointment with Dr. Google! With the advent of the Internet, there is so much medically related information available to everyone. It is inevitable that many people will attempt to self-diagnose and treat themselves. But what I observe is that most people make less-than-optimal self-doctors. Most often, people focus only on the most terrible possible diagnosis associated with a symptom and obsess about that one possibility (however rare), ignoring the long list of diagnoses that are far more likely. On the other hand, many people also ignore the most important aspects of their case as a way to delude themselves into false complacency. Guess which group of patients tends to be the worst self-diagnosticians? Ironically, in my experience,

better-educated patients are more likely to self-diagnose and to self-treat. That's a backhanded compliment, isn't it?

- **Denial.** Some people feel that if they don't go to the doctor, or if they avoid telling a doctor what's going on, then the doctor can't label them with an unwanted diagnosis. If a doctor doesn't diagnose you with anything, then maybe you're not really sick.

- **Alternative philosophies.** Many practitioners of integrative and complementary health feel that their beliefs and those of mainstream medicine do not mix well. Granted, in the past, many doctors inappropriately discounted alternative approaches. However, I believe that most doctors of the current generation are relatively comfortable with and accepting of various approaches to patient care.

- **Excessive cost.** This is a legitimate problem that not only prevents patients from accessing the American health-care system but also often prevents doctors from pursuing a diagnosis or an appropriate treatment. This is an increasingly challenging issue for all of us (but it doesn't have to be this way).

- **Too busy or stressed.** Many people are so busy with modern life that it is hard to find the time to go to the doctor, and even more difficult to comply with often time-consuming diagnostics and treatments.

- **Don't like doctors.** As hard as it is for me to believe, some people just don't like doctors! Well, you should try spending a day talking to patients! Can't we all just get along?

   Seriously, though, I get it. The charitable way to view this problem is that not every doctor is right for every patient. It's important, though, for each of us to have a dependable, competent medical team that we feel comfortable seeing, one that is available when needed.

- **The crazy, cumbersome, convoluted American health-care system got in the way.** Of course, delays aren't always the patient's fault. Doctors and other health-care practitioners, and the health-care system itself, can be the reason for delays in receiving care.

The inability to get a prompt enough appointment, unfortunately, is sometimes the reason for the delay.

In addition, the American health-care system has become exceedingly complicated and can include costly copays, prior authorizations, and odd and changing health insurance coverage for appointments, testing, and treatments. This creates significant barriers to care. Even worse, these barriers lead many people to avoid health care altogether.

As I stated, some of these reasons make lots of sense and some do not. What I don't like to see (and you won't either) is someone waiting too long to seek medical care and ending up with a tragic diagnosis that may have been treatable had they sought care sooner.

This book is intended to help you to avoid such a situation.

Bob's Cough

My father-in-law, Robert Bernat (Bob), was one of my favorite people. That's a lot to say about an in-law.

I met Bob in 1985, shortly after meeting Brenda, his oldest daughter and my future wife, and we hit it off immediately. Aspirations to medical school were quite a long way off at that time. Bob and I were kindred spirits, and we both loved his daughter. He was a friend, a mentor, and an inspirational figure for me.

Unfortunately, I also consider Bob one of my first medical cases.

I started medical school at George Washington University in the fall of 1993.

Bob apparently developed a cough during the winter of 1993–1994. He had smoked for many years. He had quit in 1990, when he met Nancy, who later became his fourth wife (yes, fourth). Nancy had noted that Bob's shirts were beginning to look a little loose at the neck.

In May 1994, Bob finally sought treatment for the cough, months after it had started. He was diagnosed with lung cancer.

I was at home on my birthday, May 17, studying for my first-year medical school finals, when Bob called to deliver the news. I remember Bob being upbeat, almost cheerful. I guess he was trying to soften the blow for us (and maybe for himself as well). It also just so happened that Brenda was three months pregnant with our daughter, Willa, at the time.

The cancer appeared to be isolated to his left lung, and there was no sign of spread. The hope back then, pretty much as it is now, was that a lung cancer is found when it is still in a location where it can be removed (a segment of a lung, or at worst the entire lung). Those cases are the ones that are likely to do better. Lung cancers that have spread to a lymph node, to the other lung, or more distant sites are more difficult to treat. Their response to chemotherapy and radiation can be poor.

Bob had his left lung removed in short order. He told us that his prognosis was decent. They had gotten it before it could spread and become more difficult to treat.

We visited Bob in June. He looked good, though it was obvious that he had lost some weight. I remember that when we greeted Bob and Nancy that day, Bob grabbed my hand rather forcefully to prevent me from slapping him on the back, where the surgeon had removed the lung and he still had a large, healing surgical wound. Another friend had done just that and caused Bob considerable pain.

We had a good visit and talked about how lucky Bob was to have caught the cancer when it was still easily treatable. We were also excited about having a child and my having completed the first year of medical school successfully. Except that Bob wasn't as lucky as we had thought.

Soon he got the news that the cancer had shown up in his right lung. Bob began chemotherapy. He had many of the common side effects from chemo, such as severe nausea and fatigue. His blood cell counts dropped at times, preventing some of his treatments. He lost his hair and a good deal of weight.

We visited with Bob in October 1994. Brenda was very pregnant by that time.

That would be our last visit with Bob. Willa was born November 27. It was a rough delivery. Brenda had hemorrhaged badly but Willa was fine, and Brenda was weak but recovering as expected. We got home from the hospital a few days later.

A few hours after we got home with our new baby and her shaky new mother, the phone rang. It was Bob and Nancy. Bob could barely speak. Half crying and half gasping, he explained that the doctors had told him that his treatments were failing. They told him he had just a month to live. Bob died just three days later. He was sixty-four years old.

Bob's cancer started as a cough. It was months before he received medical attention. Things may have been starkly different had that cough been evaluated earlier. It is my sincere hope that this book prevents as many cases like Bob's as possible.

Chapter 2

When to See the Doctor: The Cardinal Signs and Symptoms of Disease

General Rules of Thumb

Remember, the intent of *Sixty-Two Medical Complaints That Should Never Be Ignored* is not to help you diagnose and treat yourself or those around you. It is to help you decide under what circumstances, and how quickly, you need to seek medical care.

You can use the following general principles in any situation to help with that decision. *If you study and memorize anything from this book, the information in this section should be it.*

The 2-Week Rule. To be safe, any significant new symptom (that has not been previously explained), such as pain or a new cough that persists longer than 2 weeks, should be evaluated by a doctor.

The 5-Second Rule. If someone is seriously ill or hurt and needs emergency care, you should be able to make that decision in about 5 seconds. The following are tips on how to decide if someone is seriously ill or injured:

- Someone who looks ill is probably ill: no matter what the complaint, someone who is upright, smiling, and laughing, is unlikely to have an emergency. On the other hand, someone who is lying down, groaning, writhing, or otherwise appears uncomfortable; is having trouble breathing; or is confused or abnormally sleepy is likely to be seriously ill.

- Struggling to breathe: always serious.
- Shortness of breath and tiring out from the effort to breathe: always take extremely seriously.
- Loss of consciousness: always serious.
- Altered mental status, confusion: likely serious.

New Symptom Rule. Any new symptom, *not previously explained*, accompanied by any of the following, *should be considered a potential emergency until proven otherwise* and should receive prompt medical attention:

- New symptom that is severe (i.e., severe trouble breathing)
- New symptom that is very intense (i.e., intense pain)
- New symptom that involves loss of normal function (i.e., can't move, can't feel, can't think or speak, or can't see)

Previously Unexplained Symptom Rule. Any symptom not previously explained should be taken seriously. If, on the other hand, you experience a recurrence of a symptom with which you are familiar, which has previously been evaluated and explained by a physician, then you should follow the instructions you and your physician have previously discussed. If you experience a significant change in a previous symptom, such as a change in the severity or intensity or pattern of an old complaint, that should be brought to the attention of your physician.

Rapidly Changing Symptom Rule. Any new and *rapidly changing* symptom (i.e., a changing mole or lump) should prompt a call to the doctor.

Changing Skin and Bones Rule. Any significant skin change (i.e., changing rash or mole), bone abnormality (i.e., bone changing shape), or soft tissue change (i.e., swelling or lump) that is noticeable, worsening, or growing should be seen by a doctor in the near future.

Loss of Ability to Function Rule. A good rule of thumb regarding when to seek medical advice, especially when dealing with emotion- or mood-related issues (such as possible depression or anxiety), is when your symptoms become so significant that they impair your ability to function on a day-to-day basis. This might mean that you find it difficult to complete typical tasks, to function at school or at work, or to maintain basic personal relationships.

Trust Your Instincts Rule. No rule, or set of rules, explains what to do in every situation. If you are really worried about a symptom, trust your intuition and see a doctor.

Five Seconds That Seemed Like a Lifetime

It was a cold and overcast December day.

A three-month-old baby had been acting sick for a couple of days. The baby had some cold symptoms and hadn't been eating as much. Mom was concerned, so she decided that the baby shouldn't go to daycare. Instead, she brought the baby to work, which happened to be our medical office. The baby normally saw a pediatrician in the area. One of our nurses took a look at the baby and realized that he did not look well. She picked the baby up and brought him to my door.

What I saw terrified me.

The nurse was holding the baby face and belly up, with one hand under the neck and head, and the other hand under the baby's bottom. The baby's skin was gray. His arms and legs dangled loosely. He was barely moving. He was not crying.

This was the opposite of how a healthy, or even a slightly ill, baby would look. A healthy or even slightly ill baby has strong muscle tone and rosy skin, looks around, and can have a lusty cry.

In other words, using the **5-Second Rule**, we knew that this baby was extremely sick and required emergency care *immediately*! The problem was that we were in a small town many miles from the type of care that this baby might need. I understood in that instant that I was faced with a terrible dilemma.

The easy decision for me was to call 911. But I knew that if I called 911 at that moment, our local rescue squad would arrive, and because of their emergency protocols, they would take this baby to our small local hospital, which I knew did not have the facilities to treat this infant. To make matters worse, once the baby arrived at this small hospital, if the baby needed to be taken to a larger, more distant hospital (which would definitely be the case), transport protocols required that an ambulance be called from the second hospital, which could take hours. This might significantly delay necessary care. I didn't think this baby had that much time.

On the other hand, calling 911 would have been the easy thing for me to do. If anything happened to this baby while I delayed calling emergency medical services, I would most assuredly take the blame. I had a vision of a judge looking at me dubiously at my malpractice hearing.

The nurses took the infant to one of our exam rooms. A brief exam confirmed my suspicions. The baby was struggling to breathe. I instructed the staff to get our emergency kit. Supplemental oxygen was started.

I needed a plan. My thinking was that if I could find a specific hospital that could take the baby, when I called in the ambulance, I could specify where they needed to take the baby and could bypass their transportation protocol.

I went back to my office to make a phone call to the Winchester Medical Center, which was about 40 miles away. My nurses remained with the baby, with instructions to call me if his status changed. I discussed the case with an ER physician in Winchester, Virginia, who said that he would take the baby only if the neonatal team in the hospital agreed as well. I was transferred to the pediatrician on call for the hospital, which took what seemed like an eternity. That doctor refused to take responsibility for the case.

Just then, one of my nurses appeared and told me that the baby looked worse. I hurried back to the exam room. The baby was indeed struggling to breathe, even more than when I had first seen him. Staff were milling about outside the exam room door. I was sure they were wondering why I hadn't called the emergency squad. I wondered if I had made a mistake by not doing so. I asked the nurse to get out the bag and mask and prepared to begin to help the baby to breathe. I felt the weight of my decision very heavily.

Just then, a miracle occurred. As I was about to place the mask over his face, he sputtered and coughed up a mucus plug. Almost instantly, he began to breathe more easily, and his color began to improve dramatically!

I hurried back to my office again and this time called the ER at the Washington County Hospital in Hagerstown, about 25 miles away. I was lucky to get an ER doctor on the phone who was confident in his ability to take care of small infants. He told me to send him in.

We called the squad, who then came and got the baby. The plan worked. Because I had a doctor waiting for the baby in Hagerstown, they agreed to take him there. When he arrived at the ER, he was immediately intubated and placed on a ventilator. He was then transferred to Hershey Medical Center. He had a viral pneumonia that gradually improved. He was released from the hospital about a week later.

He is now a healthy teenager.

Emergency?

The family of an elderly patient called to say that she was extremely sick and was having trouble breathing. My staff told them to bring her right in and told me she was on the way. We were ready for an emergency.

Soon thereafter, my nurse knocked on my door and told me that the patient was here. I went immediately into the exam room where the patient was waiting. She greeted me, "Hi, Doctor Hahn," and smiled endearingly (I have a way with elderly female patients, by the way). She was sitting upright in one of our exam room chairs looking quite comfortable. She was breathing normally.

Even though the family had given us the impression that this would be an extreme emergency, using the **5-Second Rule**, I knew this was not an emergency at all.

If You Don't Assess Your Patients Correctly, People Might Think You're Dating Them

Adele was in her nineties. She held a special place in my heart because I had taken care of her my entire career, literally. She was the very first patient I saw when I became a practicing physician. She had come in on my first day with a head laceration, caused by falling. She needed stitches.

We got a call one afternoon that Adele wasn't feeling well. If memory serves me, she had fallen and was now somewhat confused. My nurse and I went to her home, a stately mansion unlike any other home I had seen in the area.

Adele did not seem too bad, but she appeared weak and had low blood pressure. People her age can be challenging to assess, I knew, and often don't have the reserves to fight off a significant illness or injury. I was really torn. My biggest concern was that Adele lived alone. I worried that if she fell again, or took a turn for the worse during the night, she would get into trouble before she could alert anyone. Because of that, I urged her to let me call the ambulance and have her taken to the hospital in Hagerstown, Maryland, some 25 miles to the east, where she could be more thoroughly assessed and monitored. She made it clear that she really did not want to go, though.

She argued for some time that she didn't need to go to the hospital. Her final line of reasoning was that she wouldn't have a ride home. Offhand, I told her that if she needed to get back that night, the hospital could call me and I would come get her. I only said that to get her to agree to go.

A few hours later, I was home, now in sweatpants, when I received a call from an ER nurse. She explained that Adele was ready to come home, and she had told them that I was her ride, just as I had instructed! Oh, brother!

A word about those sweatpants—they were gray when I bought them, and were made of a very light material that I loved. They quickly became my go-to lounge wear. At some point, they were in the washing machine along with something red. The sweatpants were tinged slightly pink after that. I didn't really care. I wore them at home. Also, I am secure enough in my manhood, too highly evolved, to let something like that bother me.

Wearing said sweatpants, I got in the car and drove to the hospital. Adele was in good spirits when I got there, ready to go home. It was about 7:30 in the evening by then, and Adele hadn't eaten. I suggested we get a bite to eat. Adele pointed me in the direction of the Hagerstown Sheraton (which is no longer there), which had a restaurant she liked. We took our seats in a booth. We were the only ones in the restaurant—how romantic.

A short time later, a door in the back of the restaurant, which led to a large function room, opened up. A county agency meeting of some sort was letting out, and a good number of people began to exit through the restaurant.

It turned out that Adele was a lot better connected than I knew. It seemed like almost everyone who had been attending that meeting knew Adele, and she knew them, as well. Adele introduced me to as many people as she could, "This is my doctor. He's taking me out to dinner."

I became acutely aware for the first time that it might seem a little odd that a young male doctor would take his elderly female patient out to dinner at a largely deserted restaurant late in the evening. It was then that I began to regret the choice of the pink sweatpants as well. I may not have mentioned this, but I was also wearing an old red sweatshirt.

I got the distinct impression as each of these people sized me up that they regarded me more as a poorly dressed gigolo than a doctor on a mission of mercy.

Adele was unfazed; in fact, she was delighted by the attention she was receiving. She continued to introduce me as the doctor who was taking her out to dinner.

This is one reason why it is so important to be able to effectively assess a patient in their time of need. If you get this wrong, then people may begin to think that you date your patients.

Chapter 3

General Complaints

Allergic Reaction (Anaphylaxis)
Threat Level–Anaphylaxis: HIGHEST

A severe allergic reaction, otherwise known as *anaphylaxis* (or an anaphylactic reaction), is a true medical emergency. Learning to identify the signs and symptoms of anaphylaxis and responding quickly and aggressively is crucial. The number one reason that people having an anaphylactic reaction die is failure to understand the severity of the situation. If you suspect an anaphylactic reaction, it is better to treat first and ask questions later; undertreating can kill.

A severe allergic reaction, or anaphylaxis, usually occurs rapidly, in response to common triggers that most often include insect stings, eating a particular food, or taking a medication. The most common symptoms of anaphylaxis include:

- Skin: hives, itching, swelling (swelling in the area of the mouth or tongue is especially serious)
- Breathing: difficulty breathing, wheezing
- Stomach/Gastrointestinal: abdominal pain, nausea/upset stomach, diarrhea, vomiting

The website FamilyDoctor.org describes anaphylaxis as "a life-threatening allergic reaction. It starts soon after you are exposed to something you are severely allergic to. You may have swelling, itching, or a rash with itchy bumps (hives). Some people have trouble breathing, a tight feeling in their chest, or dizziness. Some people feel anxious. Other people have stomach cramps, nausea, or diarrhea. Some people lose consciousness (pass out). A person who has anaphylaxis needs immediate medical attention."

Rapid, aggressive treatment is crucial. If someone has a known history of anaphylaxis and has medications (epinephrine, Benadryl) at home, treatment should be started immediately. In addition, phone for emergency medical care and/or go to an ER or doctor's office immediately.

Do whatever is fastest. Calling ahead to a medical facility may help, so that they are prepared to respond immediately. In my experience, this has made the difference between life and death numerous times. Treatments include:

- Epinephrine injection: Rapid injection of epinephrine ("Epi-pen") is the most important treatment that should be given immediately. Failure to give epinephrine is the most common reason that patients die. Epinephrine injection may need to be repeated after the first treatment if symptoms occur again.
- Antihistamines: Common antihistamines (H2 blockers), like Benadryl (or Allegra, Zyrtec, or Claritin) should be given, but they are not a substitute for epinephrine. Epinephrine is the first priority. Other types of antihistamines, such as Zantac or Pepcid (H1 blockers), are sometimes given as well (these are not substitutes for epinephrine either).
- Albuterol: Some patients whose breathing does not improve with epinephrine may benefit from treatment with albuterol bronchodilators.
- Steroids: Often given to prevent a second anaphylactic reaction that may occur hours after the first.

Following initial treatment, someone who had an anaphylactic reaction should be monitored closely for hours. A second-phase anaphylactic reaction can occur, even hours after the first episode.

Being prepared for an anaphylactic reaction is crucial. Any person who has a known history of an anaphylactic reaction should own at least one Epi-pen. There should be a well-known plan to respond to any anaphylactic reaction that may occur.

Excessive Thirst

Threat Level—Excessive thirst: LOW
Threat Level—Excessive thirst and a change in mental status: VERY HIGH

Excessive thirst is included in this book because it can be an important first clue that you are developing *diabetes*. The classic symptoms (which don't always occur together, by the way) of diabetes are *excessive thirst combined with excessive urination, and weight loss*. Someone who has all three symptoms at once—excessive thirst, excessive urination, and weight loss—is likely to have fairly severe diabetes.

This situation needs to be taken very seriously, *especially in children*, who are much more likely to have type 1 diabetes; their bodies do not produce insulin. Medical care needs to be started soon.

People, mostly children and young people, with new-onset type 1 diabetes can develop a syndrome known as diabetic keto-acidosis (hard to say but worse to have). Diabetic ketoacidosis is an emergency.

The most reliable indication that someone with new or untreated type 1 diabetes is in trouble, besides the symptoms already discussed, is a change in mental status (confusion, drowsiness, grogginess, lethargy, extreme sluggishness, or loss of consciousness). These people may also have a fruity breath odor. Again, this situation is an EMERGENCY, and needs to be treated immediately.

Complicating matters is that small children may not tell you something is wrong! That is why *a change in mental status* is always a very important indication.

Just so you are aware, most adults who develop diabetes have no symptoms for years. Most adults—but not all—who develop diabetes have *type 2 diabetes,* where the body does not respond properly to the insulin they produce. By the time people with type 2 diabetes develop symptoms, which may take years, the disease tends to be fairly advanced.

In my practice, the most striking example of this was a patient who had been having symptoms (excessive thirst, excessive urination, and weight loss) for over a year and had lost 60 pounds (without trying)!

Fortunately, most adults and children who are overweight will have their blood sugar (referred to as *glucose* in medical speak) checked on a regular basis as part of recommended screening. In my experience, that is how most cases of type 2 diabetes are first identified. Most of those people have no symptoms at all.

While it is less frequent, people with uncontrolled or untreated type 2 diabetes can also get into an emergency situation known as the *hyperosmolar hyperglycemic nonketotic syndrome* (really hard to say, especially when you have it). This is also an EMERGENCY.

The most reliable indication that someone with type 2 diabetes is suffering from the hyperosmolar hyperglycemic nonketotic syndrome is a change in mental status, such as confusion, excessive drowsiness, or lethargy. This is an EMERGENCY.

Fever

Threat Level—Fever: MEDIUM
Threat Level—Fever and ill or sick appearance: HIGH-VERY HIGH

In and of itself, a fever is rarely an emergency. There are some exceptions, however, which will be discussed below.

Fever is an indication that something is wrong, usually an infection, and is part of the body's response to fight against what is going on.

The first thing to know is that a fever is defined as a *body temperature over 100.4 degrees F* (or 38.0 degrees C).

Second, the height of the fever is only loosely associated with the seriousness of the illness. In other words, a very high temperature does not necessarily mean that someone is more ill than a person with a slight fever.

When is a fever an indication of a serious condition that requires medical attention?

The first rule of thumb is that when a person with a fever appears sick, they are more likely to be sick. If you have a fever but you otherwise seem comfortable, it is less likely that something is seriously wrong. On the other hand, someone with a fever who is very uncomfortable, appears to be in significant pain, is having difficulty breathing, is groaning, or is acting confused or lethargic is more likely to be seriously ill.

Call the doctor if a person with a fever has other signs (besides the fever) of a serious illness, such as:

- Fever plus a headache and stiff neck: meningitis or other serious illnesses (see section on headache)
- Fever plus a serious cough or trouble breathing: pneumonia (see section on cough)
- Fever plus a sore throat: strep throat (see section on sore throat)
- Fever plus pain with urination, more frequent urination, or back pain: urinary infection (see section on urinary symptoms)
- Fever plus severe vomiting or diarrhea
- Fever plus a rash: many diseases have a characteristic rash (see section on rashes)
- Fever plus swelling or severe pain of a joint or any other body part: infection or even cancer

Next, any person who has a fever that lasts, or comes and goes, for a period longer than a week should see a doctor.

Finally, there are a number of situations where a fever should always prompt an immediate call to the doctor or even a visit to the ER:

- Fever in any baby 0 to 30 days old
- Fever in someone who has cancer

- Fever in a person who has a weak immune system, such a person who has HIV or AIDS, or someone who is being treated for cancer or taking medications that weaken the immune system
- Fever in a person who does not have a spleen (people without a spleen have much less ability to fight certain infections)

Weight Loss, Unexplained or Unintentional
Threat Level—Weight loss, unintentional: LOW

Unexplained weight loss, that is, weight loss that occurs when we are not trying or expected to lose weight—i.e., exercising and eating less, or if you just had the stomach flu for 3 days—may be a sign of serious disease (or a miracle from God!). Unfortunately, unexplained weight loss may be a sign of cancer and can also indicate other conditions, such as diabetes (see above section on excessive thirst) or an overactive thyroid.

About once per year, a patient comes in who tells us that they have been losing weight, they have been excessively thirsty, and have been urinating excessively—for months and months! My staff knows to check that patient's blood sugar level, and the diagnosis of diabetes is made on the spot.

It is difficult to say how much unexplained loss of weight should prompt a call to the doctor. The figure that seems to be used is 5 percent of your body weight over a period of 6 to 12 months.

There are also some general rules of thumb when deciding when to call the doctor if you are experiencing unintentional weight loss:

- The more weight you are losing and the faster it is occurring, the more quickly you should contact the doctor.
- Unexplained weight loss that is combined with other symptoms, such as cough, tiredness, excessive thirst or urination, or pain, should prompt a doctor's visit.

The Right Staff

It was shortly after we opened our small practice in our small town, at about 4:30 p.m. on a Friday afternoon. We had already seen our last scheduled patient, and we were beginning to wind down.

A woman called and said that she had a history of allergic reactions to wasps and she had just been stung, and was beginning to have a reaction. My nurse told her to get to the office immediately. Fortunately, the patient's husband was there and was able to drive her in. The nurse told me that the patient was coming in, and what was going on.

We have an emergency cart that contains all the treatments necessary to take care of an allergic reaction. We got out the cart and prepared the medications she might need.

The car pulled up, and my staff met her at her car door. By that time, she was having severe difficulty breathing. She was carried into the office. She was literally moments from collapse and death. She was immediately given a shot of epinephrine. The proper dose is written on a plaque that hangs in every room of our office. A breathing treatment with albuterol was quickly started.

She recovered and did fine! Her life was saved primarily because our staff knew how to respond. They also knew enough and cared enough to meet the patient at her car (my nurse, Lindy, deserves special mention here—plus, she would kill me if I didn't mention her by name). The doctor (I) was only one part of the process that led to the patient's successful treatment. The point is that the entire medical staff (not just the doctor) can play a crucial role in a patient's care. Think about that when deciding on a medical practice.

My First On-Call in the Hospital: Thirsty Kid, Scary Night

It was my first night of hospital call on my first medical school clinical rotation, which was pediatrics. A young patient was brought to our hospital's ER because he had become confused and stuporous. The parents had noted that he had been drinking excessively and urinating more often for the past few days. Sure enough, his blood sugar level was extremely high. He had developed type 1 diabetes, the type of diabetes that more often affects children, in which glucose levels can become very high in a short period of time.

Upon first meeting our young patient, I was immediately struck by the child's odd mental status. He seemed drunk! The child's gaze was unfocused, he was slurring words, and he could barely keep his head up. There was an odd odor, as well. This was the classic fruity breath smell that reflects the body's excessive production of a substance known as ketones.

So, my first case, on my first night of call, was one of the most difficult and feared medical emergencies: diabetic ketoacidosis.

I knew it was time to worry when the resident physician I was accompanying that night said simply, "Shit!" I saw a look of what I took for extreme fear come over her face, and in turn I got scared.

I came to understand her concern as the night wore on. We began IV fluids, and then insulin, and began to construct a complicated table of blood sugar readings, sodium and potassium levels, and various calculations that we needed to update every 1 to 2 hours through the night.

Thankfully, our young patient responded well, and by the next day, we had a normally behaving and well-appearing boy.

Chapter 4

Newborns, Babies, and Infants

L et's begin with a general note of caution regarding newborns (a baby from 0 to 30 days old), babies, and infants. It can be very difficult to judge how sick a newborn, baby, or infant really is.

- Any sign of illness in a newborn (0 to 30 days old) should be taken very seriously.
- The younger the baby, the more seriously any illness should be taken.
- Any baby or infant who appears ill, very uncomfortable, or listless or who has trouble breathing should be taken very seriously.

Crying Baby That Won't Comfort
Threat Level—Crying baby that won't comfort: MEDIUM-HIGH
Threat Level—Crying baby that won't comfort and appears ill or listless or is having trouble breathing: VERY HIGH-HIGHEST

Babies cry a lot. Because of this, it is difficult to know if a baby's crying means that something is seriously wrong. However, in general, a well infant will stop crying, at least temporarily, when they are comforted. Most parents develop a set of skills, unique for their child, to comfort them.

One sign that an infant may be ill is an abnormal amount of crying, and especially crying that doesn't stop when the infant is comforted in ways that normally tend to calm them.

Diarrhea in a Baby

Threat Level—Diarrhea in a baby: MEDIUM
Threat Level—Diarrhea in a baby and the baby appears ill or has signs of dehydration: HIGH–VERY HIGH

Diarrhea is a pretty broad topic. Remember that the focus of this book is when to get to the doctor. So the focus in this section is those cases when diarrhea is cause for concern.

The first challenge is to recognize what a baby's normal stool looks like. A baby's stool is typically less solid than an adult's. Second, the color, texture, and odor can vary based on what the baby is eating or drinking. If the baby's stool becomes more watery or loose, is much more frequent than normal, or is of a much greater volume, than it is likely to be diarrhea.

The number one concern for a baby who has diarrhea is dehydration. Preventing dehydration is accomplished by increasing fluid intake—in the form of breast milk, formula, or rehydration solutions, such as Pedialyte. Do not use Gatorade, which contains too much sugar and may even worsen diarrhea.

Contact your doctor or go to the ER immediately for signs of dehydration in an infant. Signs that a baby who is having diarrhea may be becoming dehydrated include:

- Less frequent urination
- A dry appearance inside the mouth or a lack of tears when crying
- Eyes or fontanelles (the soft spots on an infant's head) that appear sunken
- A baby that is more irritable than usual or especially tired-looking or lethargic
- Dry skin or skin that remains tented up after being pinched

Also contact your doctor if your baby has diarrhea and any of the accompanying signs:

- Temperature over 100.4 in a newborn baby up to 30 days of age

- Temperature over 102 in an infant over 30 days of age
- The baby appears to be in pain
- There is blood or pus in the stool
- Severe vomiting

Fever in a Newborn

Threat Level—Fever in a newborn: VERY HIGH

First things first; we need to define a fever. *A fever is a body temperature of 100.4 degrees Fahrenheit and higher.*

In an infant, that should be a rectal temperature (sorry about that). Because of the newborn's immature immune system, the serious nature of the infections that newborns are susceptible to, and the fact that newborns are not good at telling us how they feel, newborns up to 30 days old who have a fever are considered sick until proven otherwise. They require immediate attention. However, even though this is the case, in my experience, most of these children turn out to be OK. Still, contact your doctor or go to the ER immediately—choose one where the staff is experienced with small babies.

I will elaborate on this last point because it is extremely important. In my experience, the younger the infant, the less likely you will find a doctor who is comfortable with babies' emergency care. Therefore, if you are planning to have a baby, you should plan ahead and identify a primary care doctor and a hospital where the staff are experienced and comfortable with the care of young infants.

Fever in Infants Older Than 1 Month

Threat Level—Fever in infants older than 1 month: MEDIUM
Threat Level—Fever in infants older than 1 month and infant appears ill, listless, or having trouble breathing: HIGH-VERY HIGH

Fever (rectal temperature of 100.4 degrees F and higher) in an infant over 1 month old requires a little judgment. Fever in and of itself is not an emergency. It should serve as a warning that something is wrong but taken by itself does not tell us how sick a baby is.

As a general rule, with an infant over 1 month old who has a fever, we tend to make judgments based upon how well or ill the baby looks. A well-appearing infant who is comfortable, feeding regularly, has good color, and interacts well with his/her parents is less likely to be seriously ill. An ill-appearing infant, one who seems uncomfortable, is not feeding well, who is pale or even has bluish color around the mouth (cyanosis), and is not interactive, is more likely to be seriously ill.

The height of the fever correlates with the seriousness of the illness only to a small extent. In other words, we take a higher fever more seriously, but it doesn't help much in determining the seriousness of the illness.

Another general rule is that fever of 100.4 degrees F or higher associated with the following conditions makes serious illness more likely:

- A listless or tired-appearing baby
- A crying baby that won't comfort
- A baby that has trouble breathing
- A baby with pale skin color or bluish color around the mouth or the abdomen (referred to as cyanosis)
- A baby who is having severe vomiting
- A baby with severe diarrhea (special cases, like bloody stool and currant jelly stool)
- A baby who has a serious rash

Listless or Tired-Appearing Baby

Threat Level—Listless or tired-appearing baby: VERY HIGH–HIGHEST

When trying to decide whether an infant's illness or injury is serious, one of the most worrisome findings is the baby who is lethargic and underactive or one who appears to be tiring out easily.

A well infant or one who has only a minor illness or injury will usually have a loud, lusty cry and good muscle tone. If you grab their hand or pull on their arm, they will grab back and you will feel them pull back.

A more seriously ill infant, on the other hand, may appear to be listless or lethargic, have only a weak cry, and have poor or weak muscle tone. If you hold up the infant's arm and the arm flops down weakly when you let go, that infant is more likely to be seriously ill.

Projectile Vomiting in a Baby
Threat Level—Projectile vomiting in a baby: MEDIUM-HIGH

Projectile vomiting is vomiting that is so forceful that the vomit (I'm sorry for mentioning vomit so many times in one sentence) projects, often in an arc, over a distance of up to a few feet. Projectile vomiting in a young infant may be a sign of a condition known as *pyloric stenosis.*

Pyloric stenosis is a blockage of the valve that digesting food goes through to exit the stomach (the pyloric valve). Pyloric stenosis is a relatively common condition that usually affects very young infants, typically between 3 and 5 weeks of age, and is more common in male infants and children of parents who have had the condition themselves. Pyloric stenosis is a serious condition that usually needs to be corrected surgically.

Projectile vomiting should prompt a visit to the doctor in the very near future.

Trouble Breathing in a Baby
Threat Level—Trouble breathing in a baby: VERY HIGH-HIGHEST

Trouble breathing in an infant should always be taken seriously. The difficulty is knowing what an infant who is having serious trouble breathing looks like.

First of all, even under normal circumstances, newborns and smaller infants can be notoriously irregular breathers. Healthy infants may sputter and gasp and even appear to stop breathing for a few seconds.

As a rule of thumb, a few seconds of irregular breathing should not be of concern. Irregular breathing that lasts longer than that should get your attention. The longer that irregular breathing lasts, the more concerning it becomes. Signs that your baby may be having trouble breathing can include:

- Retractions: The skin over the ribs and neck may visibly retract, or be sucked in around the bones, in someone who is struggling to breathe.
- Flaring of the nostrils.
- Breathing faster than normal: realize that infants up to one year of age may take a breath 30 to 60 times per minute, which is much faster than an adult breathes (12 to 16 breaths per minute).

There Is a Connection between Currant Jelly and Diarrhea

This is a story about currant jelly.

During my training, I was in pediatric clinic one day, working under the legendary Dr. Charles Reilly, and we saw a 4-month-old infant whose mother brought her in because she wasn't acting right.

As an aside, I should tell you a little about Dr. Reilly. He had been the chief of pediatrics in our hospital for many years but was semiretired by the time I came along. We residents knew him as the author of *The Reilly Manual*, a pocket guide to pediatrics he had compiled that to this day I keep in my office and still use as a reference.

Dr. Reilly always told us stories about the golden age of being a doctor (the 1960s and 1970s). He told us that when a doctor entered an elevator back then, everybody else got off the elevator. Also, any time the doctor walked into a nurses' station, the nurses stood and offered the doctor their chair! I trained in the 1990s, and the golden era of medicine had apparently ended.

Anyway, I digress. I'll get back to our story.

As you may remember, we had a 4-month-old baby who was "not acting right." "Not acting right" was an accurate way to describe this beautiful little baby. She was so serious. Many years later, I still remember the look she gave me. It was like, "You better figure out what's wrong here, buddy." You just couldn't get this baby to smile. She wasn't crying. She wasn't clinging to mom.

She certainly wasn't being very active. Other than that, we had little to go on. She did not have a fever. Her vital signs were normal, and her physical exam didn't provide any clues to the diagnosis. But mom's intuition felt right. Dr. Reilly and I agreed with her. Something wasn't right, but we didn't really know what the problem was. We decided to admit the baby to the hospital for observation.

Many years later, I still remember this case, as I said, because of the look on that baby girl's face, but also because we admitted the baby on what felt like relatively minor grounds. Especially in this day and age, where insurance companies and hospital utilization managers are breathing down your neck to justify every minute a patient is in the hospital, admitting a baby to the hospital because they "didn't look right" would raise many eyebrows.

A few hours later, it was early evening, and I was on the hospital's pediatric ward. Luckily, I was on call in the hospital that night so that I could follow up with the baby.

A smart nurse (thank God for them) brought the baby's diaper to show me. In the diaper was a red and purple gooey mess. The nurse gave me a knowing look. Because I was a doctor (though still in training), I understood that I was supposed to return the knowing look, which I did. I didn't know the real significance of the diaper goo, however.

A short while later, the nurse returned, and I guess she was wondering why I wasn't doing something about what she had shown me. She said something like, "Didn't that baby's stool look like currant jelly?"

Aha! She had given me the answer, only I hadn't known what the answer meant until that moment. From my studies, I knew that "currant jelly stool" was medically synonymous with the diagnosis of intussusception. The problem was that I had never seen currant jelly before (much less a case of intussusception)! Have you ever had currant jelly? Would you know currant jelly if you saw it?

If the answer is no, then right now, Google "currant jelly images" and familiarize yourself with the appearance of currant jelly. I'm serious. Intussusception is a very serious condition, especially common in infants, where one part of the bowel "telescopes" inside another section of the bowel downstream, causing an intestinal blockage. It is a serious condition that, left untreated, can be deadly.

There are two ways to treat a serious case. The first, less invasive, treatment is to administer a barium enema, in the hopes that the pressure of the enema will force the "telescoped" portion of the bowel back into position. You use barium because it shows up on an x-ray and enables visualization of the bowel. We tried this, but it was unsuccessful.

The next option was surgery. We actually imported a pediatric surgeon from a university hospital about an hour away. There was great fanfare, as this was a relatively rare case in our hospital. A number of residents, and the chief of pediatrics, scrubbed in to observe, and we even photographed the procedure.

Our young patient did fine, and she was discharged home a few days later. So the lesson here is that diarrhea that looks like currant jelly is a sign of a serious condition, "intussusception."

Next time you encounter currant jelly, maybe you'll think of this case! Yum! Bon appetit!

Pale Newborn Needs Spaghetti Tongs

I had been in practice for about 9 months. My practice was located in the small western Maryland town of Hancock, and my wife, daughter, and I lived nearby in beautiful Berkeley Springs, West Virginia.

It was 5:30 in the morning. I had just gotten up and was about to leave the house to go running. It was still dark outside. Suddenly, I began to hear a car's horn. Headlights were coming up the driveway.

It was Bob and Jen, good friends whom we had met years earlier when we lived in Washington, DC. They now lived in West Virginia as well. We ran into them at a drumming circle, of all things, soon after our move. Shortly thereafter, Jen had become pregnant. Maybe it had happened after the drumming circle!

Jen was due in late March. She planned to deliver the baby in Kensington, Maryland, about two hours away.

As her pregnancy progressed, we joked about what to do if the baby came early. I had even planned to make sure I had access to an emergency delivery kit, just in case the baby came during the winter and Bob and Jen got stuck in the snow. Of course, the odds of anything like that were low. I had delivered lots of babies during my residency training but was no longer doing deliveries now that I was in practice.

One night in late March, Jen went into labor. They called our friend, Genesee, who was to serve as their delivery assistant. They all got into Bob and Jen's car, with their young son, Dakota, as well, and started the drive to Maryland. They had not gone very far when they realized things had progressed too quickly, and the baby's delivery was imminent.

They tried to call my house, but in a very odd and rare turn of events, our phone was off the hook. They bypassed our local hospital, heading for our home.

They did not make it. Baby boy Lassa was born in the parking lot of a hair salon a couple of miles from our house. Genesee performed the delivery. They wrapped the baby in Jen's dress and continued on their way to our home. The placenta was still intact, and Lassa was still attached to the umbilical cord.

I went out to investigate, and seeing who it was and quickly discerning what had happened, I ushered Jen into the house. The first room off our front door was our new dining room, where I had just installed a wood floor. This room had been transformed from what had initially been a garage, first into an art studio by the previous owners, and then into our brand new dining room (by me).

Jen looked shaky, so I gallantly pulled our futon couch to the middle of the room, so that she wouldn't have to walk as far. Moving the futon made a large scratch in my new wood floor! It's still there to this day. But hey, it's just a floor! What does a brand new floor matter—that you had labored over for so many hours, and had then fixed and painted the walls, and then repainted the walls because the first color was atrocious—what does that matter when a new baby has entered the world? There's no comparison, right? That scratch doesn't bother me at all! It doesn't!

I did a quick assessment of the baby and thought he looked pale and was being a little too quiet. That could mean that he was losing blood through the umbilical cord. We would need to clamp and cut the cord as soon as we could. But I couldn't quite figure out what I had at home to do that with.

Then it came to me: spaghetti tongs! I called to my wife, Bibi, to get our spaghetti tongs, which served as an adequate clamp for the moment.

As many of you readers probably know, the real answer is shoelaces. Lots of my smarty-pants outdoorsy female friends have told me that the answer is shoelaces. You tie the cord in two places and then cut in the middle.

Soon, the rescue squad arrived. I didn't know they had been called.

Fortunately, the squad had medical equipment, and we clamped the cord properly The baby looked good.

Then, we set about delivering the placenta, which came after a short time and with a gush of blood (which got on my futon and the new floor).

Lassa is now a healthy young man whom I recently beat in arm wrestling. Maybe he should fix my floor.

Chapter 5

The Head

Headache

Threat Level—Headache: LOW–MEDIUM
Threat Level—Headache and *high fever, visible discomfort, or ill appearance:*
VERY HIGH
Threat Level—Severe headache or headache and signs of stroke:
VERY HIGH–HIGHEST

Headaches are a very common complaint. Their severity can range from mildly annoying to intense and debilitating.

Headaches can occur for many reasons. A headache may occur with no apparent cause and not relate to any serious condition. On the other hand, a headache may be the first symptom of a serious condition, such as meningitis, a bleed into the brain, or a brain tumor.

It would be beyond the scope of this book to discuss the causes and diagnosis of every type of headache or headache syndrome. Our purpose when it comes to headaches is to explain when you need to contact the doctor in a timely manner because early diagnosis and treatment may prevent serious consequences.

As a general rule, new onset of headaches should be taken seriously. That is, if you begin to experience headaches and have never had headaches in the past or on a regular basis, then you should consult a physician.

For people who tend to suffer from headaches on a regular basis, a change in the pattern of the headaches should be taken seriously. Many people experience headaches, such as migraine headaches or tension headaches, on a regular basis. For chronic headache sufferers, a change in the pattern of the headaches' frequency, intensity, location, or the other symptoms usually associated with the headaches should prompt a call to the doctor.

Headache Red Flags

Threat Level—Worst headache of your life: HIGHEST
Threat Level—Headache and *high fever, visible discomfort, or ill appearance:*
VERY HIGH

Doctors are taught that there are a number of headache "red flags" that are indications that a headache may be more serious, and should receive medical attention promptly. According to an article in the February 2001 issue of *American Family Physician,* they include:

- Headaches that begin to occur for the first time in a patient over the age of 50
- Sudden, severe headache
- The worst headache of your life (signals a bleed in the brain, a subarachnoid hemorrhage, until proven otherwise)
- Headaches that are occurring more often over time
- Headaches that are becoming more severe over time
- Headaches associated with signs of illness, such as fever, stiff neck, a rash, or joint pain
- Headaches associated with loss of vision or change in vision, or numbness, weakness, or loss of function of an arm or leg
- Headaches in a patient who has cancer or HIV infection
- Headaches that begin after trauma to the head
- Headaches that are triggered by strenuous exercise or exertion
- Headaches that awaken you from sleep
- New-onset headaches in a pregnant woman

One-Sided Headache in a Person Over the Age of 50
Threat Level—One-sided headache in a person over the age of 50: MEDIUM-HIGH

One headache syndrome, which tends to occur in older people, bears special mention because prompt diagnosis and treatment may prevent blindness. Giant cell arteritis (GCA), also known as temporal arteritis, is a type of vasculitis, or inflammation of the blood vessels, that causes headaches in people who are usually over the age of 50. Left untreated, GCA can cause blindness or even death. Prompt treatment with steroids provides almost immediate relief.

Typically, GCA begins with a headache that affects only one side of the head, usually located in the temple, or over the ear, and is accompanied by tenderness of the scalp in those areas. In other words, you may feel pain if you press on the area where the headaches are occurring.

Time is of the essence in GCA, so evaluation and treatment should take place as quickly as possible.

When His Headache Was Worse, His Tongue Went to the Right

Truth be told, one of the hardest things about evaluating modern patients complaining of pain is being able to decipher who is telling the truth and who is making their pain up in order to get a prescription for narcotics. Believe it or not, doctors don't have a magic test that enables them to tell the difference.

The patient was a middle-aged male wearing a red, white, and blue bandana, a leather jacket, and torn jeans. He was unshaven. He looked like a cross between a biker and a pirate (I don't have anything against either, by the way). He had a reputation, according to my staff, for abusing and selling narcotics.

He came in complaining that he was having increasingly severe headaches over the past few days. The headache was located at the back of his head. He noted that the intensity of the pain waxed and waned, but when the pain was most intense, his tongue involuntarily moved to the right. I thought that was an impressive complaint. I had not heard that before, and I have not heard it since.

Unfortunately, the patient also exhibited some of the signs that can indicate that a patient is seeking drugs (and not telling the truth). He cursed aggressively a number of times throughout the appointment, "You need to give me something for this fucking pain!" He also asked specifically for Percocet (a well-known narcotic).

My memory of the exact progression of the proceeding events is a little foggy, but I am sure that I did not give the patient Percocet during that first appointment. But I was on call that week and received a message from the patient a couple of days later. His severe headaches persisted. An MRI of his head was ordered. Again, I resisted his requests for Percocet.

Then, on Friday evening, he called again. He reiterated his story and demanded Percocet. I was truly torn. Many drug-seeking patients come in on Friday to get drugs for the weekend. On the other hand, he had contacted me a third time, and his story was concerning.

I got him a prescription for Percocet.

The MRI showed that the patient had a rare type of brain tumor that turned out to be cancerous.

At that point, with a serious diagnosis and an obvious and legitimate cause of his pain, I began to write him Percocet prescriptions on a regular basis.

He admitted to me later that he was selling some of those prescriptions rather than taking the medication! Live and learn!

Headache and Fever

I was on call in the hospital one Sunday during my residency. Shortly after my shift had started, I received a call from a man complaining of a headache and fevers. He told me that he had been having the headaches for a few days and had spoken to one of my colleagues on call a few days earlier. The headaches were fairly intense, and he was concerned that he was not improving, as well as that he continued to have fevers.

I was concerned that he could have meningitis, but based on the fact that he sounded well over the phone, and that he had not gotten more ill over this time period, he was more likely to have *viral* meningitis than the dreaded *bacterial* meningitis. If he had had bacterial meningitis, he would have been much more ill.

I told him to continue to rest, to get extra fluids, to take something for the headache, and to call me back or come to the ER if he felt he was worsening.

A few hours later, I received a call from a doctor in the hospital's ER. The patient with the headache had come to the ER. He walked into the ER on his own. He lay down on a gurney, and shortly thereafter, became unconscious. He never regained consciousness.

A CAT scan of his head showed multiple tumors that had hemorrhaged into the brain. His white blood cell count was extremely high, indicating that he had acute leukemia. The tumors in his brain were from the leukemia. He died overnight.

I was wracked with guilt that I had not brought the patient to the ER more quickly. The fact is, though, that nothing could have been done at that point. That morning, I spent some time speaking to the patient's wife, discussing the case and expressing my condolences. About a week later, I received a call from her. I was concerned that she was calling because she was angry with me (and would be threatening to sue me, of course).

In fact, she was calling not out of anger, but out of concern for me. I had seemed very upset after her husband's death, and she just wanted to make sure I was OK. One of the remarkable aspects of practicing medicine is that now and then patients do as much (or more) for me as I do for them.

Chapter 6

The Eyes

Eyes are important. Even though we have two of them, it is best to protect them both. Early identification and treatment of a serious eye condition may save your eyesight, so knowing the symptoms of an eye-related emergency is crucial. There are four eye-related symptoms that should always prompt a call to the doctor:

- Significant pain of the eye(s)
- Sudden changes in vision
- Sudden loss of vision
- Significant change in the appearance of the eye(s) or eyelid(s), such as eye redness or swelling

Change in the Appearance of the Eye(s) or Eyelid(s)
Threat Level—Change in the appearance of the eye(s) or eyelid(s): MEDIUM–HIGH
Threat Level—Significant change in the appearance of the eye(s) accompanied by eye pain or change in vision: HIGH

Certain changes in the appearance of the eye should always receive medical attention. A bulging eye, sudden crossed eyes, or a wandering eye, a condition where one eye's movement does not match the movement of the other, should receive immediate medical attention.

Eye redness, known in medical circles as the "red eye," is a very common medical complaint. There are many causes of a red eye, many of which are not so serious (pink eye, which is usually a mild viral infection, allergies, or dry eyes), and some of which are quite serious (bacterial infections, injuries).

Of note, one of the causes of a red eye that frightens patients the most (because it looks so bad), the subconjunctival hemorrhage (see Image 1), is actually not serious at all. In a subconjunctival hemorrhage, the white part of the eye (the sclera) develops a sudden blood-red appearance, usually affecting only part of the sclera, though rarely it can affect the entire white of the eye (on the other hand, if the redness affects the pupil, that is an entirely different problem that needs immediate medical attention). The appearance of a subconjunctival hemorrhage can be quite impressive, and that is what prompts people to call the doctor. There are usually few other symptoms. There is usually no pain. The condition results from minor trauma, and most often, patients can't point to a specific incident as the cause. There is no treatment necessary. It looks serious, but it is not.

A red eye should prompt a call to the doctor when it is accompanied by:

- A change in vision or loss of vision
- Significant eye pain, headache, or sensitivity to light
- A gritty sensation or the sensation that something is in the eye, especially if there is a possible exposure to a foreign body
- Significant swelling of the eye or eyelid
- A red eye that doesn't improve after 2 to 3 days

A sty (see Image 2) is also a very common problem that affects the eye. A sty is an infection of the eyelid and can affect the edge of the eyelid or the inside of the eyelid.

A sty usually begins with a small pimple or lump on or near the edge of the eyelid. It can grow and become painful. A sty is usually treated with warm compresses in the hopes that it will open and drain. You should see your doctor for a sty that causes significant pain, is associated with a change in vision, or one that does not resolve on its own after 3 to 5 days.

Pain of the Eye
Threat Level—Eye pain: HIGH (It's your eye!)

Pain in and around the eye may have an obvious cause, such as an injury or foreign body, but may also be the first symptom of a serious infection or a serious disease, such as glaucoma. Note that people who wear contact lenses, or who have recently undergone eye surgery, should always treat significant pain of the eye as an emergency. People who have glaucoma should treat significant eye pain as an emergency as well.

In addition, eye pain associated with the following conditions should receive immediate medical care:

- Eye pain accompanied by a change in vision or sensitivity to light
- Eye pain accompanied by redness or discharge from the eye
- Severe eye pain following an injury to the eye
- Eye pain in a person who has been working around wood or metal products that could get into the eye
- Eye pain after welding or following a chemical splash

Sudden Changes in Vision
Threat Level—Sudden vision changes: HIGH-VERY HIGH

Sudden changes in vision, even in the absence of eye pain, can be an indication of a serious eye condition. For instance, the appearance of flashes of light or visual floaters may be a sign of a detached retina. Visual halos may be a sign of glaucoma. Contact your physician promptly if you experience any of the following vision changes:

- Blurred vision
- Flashes of light
- Floaters (spots, strings, cobwebs, shadows that obscure vision)

- Halos of light
- Double vision

Sudden Loss of Vision
Threat Level–Sudden loss of vision: HIGHEST

Any sudden loss of vision is a true eye emergency. Partial visual loss or full loss of vision should be evaluated immediately.

Chapter 7

Ears, Nose, and Throat

EARS
Ear Pain
Threat Level—Ear pain: MEDIUM

The vast majority of ear pain cases turn out to be minor problems. However, the ear is a rich organ that can develop a veritable bouquet of nuanced problems, some of which can actually, even if only rarely, kill you.

And let's not forget: untreated or inappropriately diagnosed and treated ear conditions might lead to deafness, which is an important problem.

Still, we need to talk about ear infections (otitis media and otitis externa). And the discussion about ear infections is as much about *not doing anything* as it is about doing something—such as treatment with antibiotics.

The 1990s were, for many of us, a great time to be alive. Sure, we had our problems, but remember how much sense everything seemed to make back then compared to now? Didn't life seem much simpler somehow?

Things were so great that the 1990s were the decade of the child's ear infection. Because of the standard children's vaccines that had come along in the period roughly between 1960 and 1990, most serious children's diseases, the ones that actually killed thousands of children every year in the time before vaccines, were largely gone. American doctors from my generation (I began my training in 1993) never saw cases of measles or polio. We see so few cases of chickenpox that grandmothers tend to be better diagnosticians of chickenpox than doctors of my era.

Things had become so good by the 1990s that we were just cleaning up around the edges of children's infectious disease, treating issues like sore throats, runny noses—and ear infections.

It was the epic medical clash of the 1990s (and early 2000s). Moms demanded antibiotics. They even knew which antibiotics worked best (amoxicillin, the pink stuff). But doctors were being taught that antibiotics were being overused, and studies from Europe showed that most children with ear infections didn't even require antibiotics to get better.

I remember going toe-to-toe with more than a few moms on this issue. It was a battle that seemed to take place at least a few times per day. I was even counseled, at one point, by one of my faculty members that "it never pays to go toe-to-toe with a mom." But it was the right thing to do (and so I did it)!

Fortunately, with the advent of the pneumonia vaccine that we began to give babies in the year 2000, even ear infections have faded substantially from the usual tableau of childhood infectious diseases (the pneumonia vaccine eliminated many varieties of the bacterium *Streptococcus pneumoniae*, which caused a large percentage of ear infections).

When to Go to the Doctor for Ear Infections

All that being said, it is certainly appropriate to bring to the doctor any child who is complaining of significant ear pain, especially if they are showing other signs of illness, such as a high fever.

First and foremost, there is more than one cause of ear pain. Only by examining a patient's ear can a diagnosis of an ear infection be made (otitis media, an infection behind the ear drum, is the most common type, followed by otitis externa, or "swimmers ear," an infection of the ear canal).

Infants under 6 months of age showing significant signs of illness (they won't tell you their ear hurts), such as a fever or significant discomfort, should be evaluated as quickly as possible. I would usually recommend that they be seen the day they begin to show signs of illness.

Children over 6 months of age should be seen if they are having severe pain or high fever (102.2 degrees F or higher). It is appropriate to treat a child's ear infection with antibiotics in the following instances, according to the American Academy of Pediatrics:

- All children less than 6 months of age with an ear infection.
- Children over 6 months of age with severe pain or fever of 102.2 degrees F or higher.
- Children between 6 months and 2 years of age with an infection in both ears.

Other children, those 6 months of age or older who do not have severe pain or high fever, can be observed, as long as there is a plan to treat any child who does not improve over 2 to 3 days.

Other Causes of Ear Pain

While typical infections, otitis media and otitis externa, are the most common causes of ear pain in children, there are other less common infections, as well as non-infection-related causes of ear pain (which become more common in adults).

Malignant otitis externa is a severe type of ear infection that most commonly occurs in people with uncontrolled diabetes or who are immunosuppressed. Mastoiditis is an infection that extends to the mastoid bone, the bony prominence that can be felt just behind the ear, and usually occurs in untreated or undertreated otitis media.

Noninfection causes of ear pain can include foreign bodies in the ear (I love to look in an ear to see that something is looking back at me—that's right, we find bugs from time to time, but also popcorn, BBs, etc.), shingles inside the ear (a problem known as Ramsay Hunt syndrome, which I first heard discussed on the TV show *ER*), and growths, such as the cholesteatoma (a destructive growth that can develop behind the middle ear).

So how quickly should an adult with ear pain be seen by their doctor? The severity of the pain and other accompanying symptoms should be used as a guide. You should be seen as soon as possible for:

- Severe ear pain
- Ear pain accompanied by loss of hearing
- Ear pain accompanied by a fever
- Ear pain accompanied by swelling or redness of the ear
- Ear pain accompanied by facial paralysis or a change in vision

Persistent ear pain, even if it is not severe, and even if it is not accompanied by any of the symptoms listed above, should be evaluated within 1 to 2 weeks.

Ringing in the Ears (Pulsatile Tinnitus)
Threat Level—Ringing in the ears (pulsatile): MEDIUM

Tinnitus, or ringing in the ears, is very common and rarely serious. That does not mean that it is not annoying to those who experience it. It also happens to be annoying to physicians because there is rarely anything we can do about it. But we don't hold that against you.

One type of tinnitus, however, should usually be evaluated, even though it still only rarely represents a serious underlying condition; it is called pulsatile tinnitus. There are two types of tinnitus: nonpulsatile and pulsatile. Pulsatile tinnitus is ringing in the ears, usually only "heard" in one ear, where the noise (usually described as a ringing, buzzing, a high- or low-pitched humming, or even a roaring sound) pulses with the heartbeat.

Pulsatile tinnitus can be a sign of a serious condition, such as an aneurysm or blockage of an artery that supplies blood to the head and brain.

How quickly should you see the doctor? If pulsatile tinnitus is accompanied by a headache, dizziness, or any other neurological change, such as a change in vision or weakness or numbness in an arm or leg, evaluation should take place as soon as possible.

In the absence of these symptoms, pulsatile tinnitus should likely receive medical attention if it persists for more than 1 to 2 weeks.

Sudden Hearing Loss
Threat Level–Sudden hearing loss: HIGH

This is important. Sudden hearing loss is an "urgency" (urgency implies that medical care must happen as quickly as possible, but it is not an emergency that requires driving through red lights to get to the ER). The more quickly it is treated, the more likely you are to recover your hearing, though.

Sudden sensorineural hearing loss (SSHL), or sudden deafness, which is unexplained rapid hearing loss, usually in one ear, needs to be diagnosed and treated with steroids quickly, within 1 to 3 days, but the sooner the better. Steroids that are started after one month are unlikely to help. The hearing loss is usually noted over a short period of time, usually less than 3 days. SSHL-related hearing loss is often noted upon awakening.

If you experience sudden hearing loss, you should try to be seen by your doctor that same day if possible.

NOSE

Nosebleeds
Threat Level–Nosebleeds: SEE BELOW

Nosebleeds are rarely an emergency, but any significant bleeding (from any part of the body, including the nose) can be an emergency under the following circumstances:

- There is a large amount of blood loss that does not stop after 15 to 20 minutes of treatment (applying pressure).
- There is enough blood loss to begin feeling the effects (weakness, lightheadedness, pale skin color, chest pain, or shortness of breath).

- There is a known disorder of coagulation, the body's ability to stop bleeding (this includes taking a blood-thinning medication, such as warfarin, or having a condition such as hemophilia, von Willebrand's disease, and others).
- You have a nosebleed following nasal surgery or an injury that includes significant facial trauma.
- You have very high blood pressure.

By far the bigger issue when it comes to nosebleeds is to know the proper method of treatment. The typical approach used (that is incorrect) is to tilt the head back or to lie down, and to stuff the nose with wads of tissue. Proper treatment of a nosebleed includes:

- Sitting upright with the head slightly forward.
- Pinching the soft end of the nose firmly between two fingers for 10 minutes.
- If the bleeding does not stop after 10 minutes, repeat for another 10 minutes.

The other issue is to identify the cause of the nosebleed, which becomes important if someone experiences a number of nosebleeds in a short amount of time. Common causes include very dry air, a recent cold virus or allergies, and frequent use of medications such as aspirin or nonsteroidal anti-inflammatory drugs (NSAIDs: ibuprofen, naproxen, etc.), especially when any of these conditions are combined with nose picking (though no one in *my* practice ever picks their nose, apparently).

THROAT

Throats do two things that let you know there is a problem: they hurt and they swell. Throats also turn various colors, which gives you a clue as to what's going on, but it's usually the pain that gets you to look in the first place.

While throat pain is the way that the throat usually lets you know you have a problem, it is swelling that tells you that you may have an emergency. Significant swelling of the throat is an emergency because it may block your airway. In other words, swelling of the throat may make it difficult, or even impossible, to breathe.

Fortunately, because of childhood vaccinations (the Hib vaccine), my generation of American physicians very rarely sees one of the most dreaded throat infections, epiglottitis (I have never seen a case, thankfully). Epiglottitis can cause severe swelling of the throat (the epiglottis) and used to be a common pediatric emergency. Thank you, childhood vaccinations.

Abscess of the Throat or Neck

Threat Level—Abscess of the throat or neck: HIGH-VERY HIGH
Threat Level—Abscess of the throat or neck and *trouble breathing or swallowing: VERY HIGH-HIGHEST*

Throat and neck infections can lead to abscess formation (an abscess is an infection characterized by swelling due to an accumulation of pus).

The swelling associated with an abscess of the throat or neck can block the airway, so this needs to receive medical attention as soon as possible.

Mononucleosis

Threat Level—Mononucleosis: LOW-MEDIUM
Threat Level—Mononucleosis and *sore throat causing trouble breathing or swallowing: VERY HIGH-HIGHEST*

Mononucleosis is a well-known viral infection that tends to afflict teenagers and young adults. Also known as the "kissing disease," mononucleosis is usually a relatively mild infection, causing a flulike illness and tiredness. In rare cases, mono can be quite serious, however.

The reason that mononucleosis is mentioned in this section is that many kids suffering from mono will have a pretty bad sore throat. These children should be monitored closely because, in some instances, the sore throat can be severe, and significant throat swelling can occur.

One of my pediatric faculty members, the legendary Dr. Reilly, made sure each of his medical students knew the stories of two of his teenage patients, both of whom died from suffocation as a result of throat swelling caused by mononucleosis. This is why I always take these patients seriously.

Strep Throat
Threat Level—Strep throat: MEDIUM

In children, the most common serious cause of a sore throat is strep throat, an infection with the Group A beta hemolytic strep (GABHS) bacteria. There are many varieties of strep bacteria (Group A, B, C, etc.), but it is infection specifically with the Group A beta hemolytic strep that concerns us here.

GABHS is serious because, if left untreated, this particular variety of strep throat infection can go on to cause rheumatic fever, a very serious condition that can cause damage to the heart. *Prompt treatment, antibiotics given within 9 days of the start of a GABHS infection, prevents this dreaded complication.*

Rarely, GABHS throat infection can also go on to cause serious kidney problems (post-streptococcal glomerulonephritis), which can lead to kidney failure. Even though this is rare, it cannot be prevented by antibiotic treatment of strep throat. But this is another reason that it is important that children with strep throat get treatment *promptly*, to prevent spread of infection to others (who could then develop rheumatic fever or post-streptococcal glomerulonephritis).

Strep throat is most common in children aged 4 to 16, and most commonly presents with sore throat and fever, and maybe a red rash (scarlet fever), and the *absence* of symptoms of the common cold, such as runny nose and cough.

When to see the doctor for throat pain:

- Throat pain associated with signs of significant throat swelling is a true emergency. Patients should be kept as calm as possible. Do not try to look in the throat with a tongue depressor because this may cause the throat to go into spasm. Signs of significant throat swelling include:
  - Intense pain.
  - Difficulty breathing.
  - Hot potato voice: A hot potato voice sounds muffled or garbled, as if the person is trying to talk with a hot potato in their mouth.
  - Drooling.
  - Inability to swallow.
  - The tripod position: People with significant neck or throat swelling who are having trouble breathing will often lean forward, with the neck extended and arched backwards, in an effort to keep the airway open.
- Strep throat: Children with strep throat should be seen as soon as possible because they are relatively contagious, but I wouldn't consider this an emergency. Treatment needs to begin within 9 days to prevent progression to rheumatic fever. Of note, children are considered infectious until they have been on antibiotics for 24 hours and have no fever.
- Mononucleosis: Teenagers and young adults who may have mononucleosis and have a severe sore throat should be monitored closely. Again, this is not usually an emergency, but they should be seen as soon as possible and monitored closely for difficulty breathing or swallowing.
- Other throat or neck pain: Even in the absence of obvious swelling or other signs of illness, throat or neck pain or hoarseness that does not get better after 3 to 4 weeks should be checked by a doctor.

Picking My Nose Broke My Mother's Back

I am not proud of this, but I use this story in my practice so that others might learn from my mistakes. As a child, I was a nose picker. There, I said it. The first step toward fixing some problems is admitting that you have one in the first place.

Sometime around fifth or sixth grade, I began to have frequent nosebleeds.

I don't remember the nosebleeds being particularly severe. It was the frequency of the bleeds that became annoying (to my mother). My mother took me to our family doctor, the great Dr. Simeon Siegel. He explained that most nosebleeds were caused by nose picking. He asked me if I picked my nose. How dare he suggest such a thing! I was horrified that I was accused of such low behavior. My mother, of course, had seen me do it hundreds of times and had yelled at me just as often. Still, it was the principle. I feigned innocence.

Dr. Siegel taught us the proper way to treat nosebleeds and gave me tubes of Neosynephrine, a gel that was supposed to stop the bleeding. The nosebleeds persisted.

I was then sent to an ear-nose-throat (ENT) specialist. I was pleased because this got me out of school for the day. It was a cold winter day.

The ENT also accused me of being a nose picker! I continued to deny. He cauterized my nose with a silver nitrate stick, which was fairly irritating, as I remember.

Outside of the ENT office there was ice on the steps. My mother slipped and fell. The fall broke a vertebra in her back. She had bouts of minor back pain for the rest of her life.

Nose picking can break your mother's back. Don't pick your nose.

The Ears, They Are A-Ringing

This is the story of what may be my most brilliant diagnosis and medical advice ever. Like everyone else, I have my good days, and I have days that aren't that good. On this day, I believe that I made a diagnosis that no other doctor would have made. Well, maybe that's going a little far, but it's OK to suffer, at least now and then, with delusions of medical grandeur. Anyway, it's good to be confident (but not overconfident) when you practice a profession where people's lives are on the line.

The patient complained of ringing in the ears—otherwise known as tinnitus. On the surface, this case didn't seem like it was going to be particularly interesting, at least at first. Tinnitus is rarely serious. To make matters worse, we rarely identify a specific cause, and there is rarely anything significant that we can do to make the problem go away. I am a firm believer that a thorough history is the best way to get to the answer to any medical conundrum.

"How long has this been going on?" I asked the patient.

"A couple of weeks," he answered.

I continued, "Do you always hear the ringing, or is it only at certain times?" The patient answered, "You know, it only bothers me when I listen to music." I figured that the patient must be listening to loud heavy metal music. Exposure to loud noise is a common trigger for tinnitus. "What music have you been listening to?" I asked.

"Bob Dylan" was his reply. That's folk music, though, the opposite of heavy metal.

I have listened to a fair amount of Bob Dylan music myself. An idea occurred to me.

"Have you been listening to John Wesley Harding?" I asked. John Wesley Harding was a late 1960s Dylan album. It marked a return to his folk music roots, after he had a recorded a number of famed "electric" albums.

"That's amazing! How did you know?" the patient exclaimed.

I knew because I had listened to the album many times myself, and the harmonica on that album can be so grating at times (no offense to Bob Dylan—I love Bob) that you have to turn it down, even though the vocals and other music sound just fine. It was the strangest diagnosis and medical advice I had ever given.

"Your problem is Bob Dylan. Stop listening to Bob Dylan and the ringing in your ears will go away." I advised.

He got better.

Chapter 8

Chest/Cardiovascular System

Abnormal Heartbeat

Threat Level–Abnormal heartbeat: LOW–MEDIUM
Threat Level–Abnormal heartbeat and chest pain, difficulty breathing,
dizziness, weakness, or otherwise not feeling well: VERY HIGH–HIGHEST

The heartbeat can be abnormal in three ways:

- Too fast
- Too slow
- Irregular

Palpitations are a sensation of an abnormal heartbeat. In an adult, the normal heart beats 60 to 100 times per minute—though a little slower or a little faster may be normal—in a very regular rhythm. Infants and smaller children have a faster heart rate.

As with many of the issues discussed in this book, an abnormal heartbeat may be of little consequence, or it may represent a life-threatening emergency. Fortunately, there is a simple rule of thumb that should guide you in deciding whether an abnormal heartbeat needs to be evaluated by a doctor. An abnormal heartbeat may be serious if it is associated with any of the following:

- Chest pain
- Difficulty breathing
- Dizziness, lightheadedness, or fainting

In general, the more intensely you experience the associated symptoms, the more likely it is that an abnormal heartbeat is serious, and the more quickly you should seek medical attention.

As a second rule of thumb, if you feel that your heartbeat is abnormal and this has not been evaluated by a doctor in the past (and the cause is known), it should be checked in the near future.

Chest Pain

Threat Level—Chest pain: VERY HIGH–HIGHEST

This is the big one, Elizabeth!

Understanding the significance of chest pain is one of the most important issues in all of medicine. Chest pain is the most common symptom of a heart attack or a signal that you are about to have a heart attack, and heart attacks and heart disease are the number one killers in America.

Chest pain can also indicate a number of other medical issues, some of which are very serious, like a pulmonary embolism (blood clot in the lungs), and some of which not so much, like costochondritis (pain of the chest wall).

The classic symptoms of a heart attack include chest pain—"angina"—that lasts more than a few minutes, plus:

- Pressure, squeezing, or fullness in the chest
- Difficulty breathing
- Sweating
- Nausea

The pain of a heart attack may also be felt in the neck or jaw, or one (usually the left) or both arms.

The pain of a heart attack may be triggered by physical exertion or a stressful experience.

Receiving medical care quickly when you are having a heart attack, or when you are about to have one, is crucial because today we have the ability to stop, or even prevent, damage to the heart. I believe that what we do for hearts today is one of the great modern miracles of science and medicine.

But, as we like to say, "Time is muscle." The heart is a muscle, and the sooner a heart attack is treated, the less muscle damage occurs.

Unfortunately, heart attacks rarely present with all of the classic symptoms. Women's symptoms can be especially tricky to interpret (women are special!).

So how do we know which of the patients having chest pain are actually having a heart attack or are at high risk for having one? A number of heart attack risk factors help us make the decision. The more risk factors a patient has, the more likely it is that the chest pain could be a sign of a serious condition.

Risk factors that increase the likelihood of heart disease, or a heart attack, include:

- Having a previous diagnosis of heart disease or a heart attack
- Being a man (men have higher risk than women, but women are catching up)
- Older age
- Smoking
- Heart disease or heart attacks running in the family (especially a parent or sibling)
- High blood pressure
- High cholesterol
- Diabetes
- Being overweight or obese
- Lack of physical activity and an unhealthy diet
- High-stress lifestyle (especially unemployment)

No single risk factor is more important than another. Doctors are taught to look at the pattern of the chest pain (the classic pattern is described above) and then to factor in any and all of the risk factors to determine the likelihood of heart disease or a heart attack.

So, how do you decide if chest pain is serious? Keep it simple. Seek immediate care for chest pain if:

- There is no obvious cause of chest pain other than heart disease or a heart attack.
- If you have any of the risk factors named above.

People's Pharmacy!

I used to listen every Saturday morning to the syndicated radio program *The People's Pharmacy*. I would even call in to the program every now and then, usually to argue with one of the show's guests.

One Saturday, the featured guest was Dr. Barry Sears, the famed developer of *The Zone Diet*. A man called in to the show interested in Dr. Sears's views on the use of statin cholesterol-lowering medications. He said that his doctor had placed him on a statin. He reviewed his cholesterol panel numbers with the good doctor. I am paraphrasing here, but Dr. Sears's response was something like "Your doctor doesn't know what he's talking about."
There was something that bothered me about this conversation. I couldn't put my finger on what it was, though. I went about my morning and soon became consumed by other thoughts, forgetting about *The People's Pharmacy* and Dr. Sears.

Of course, I have conversations about statins almost every day with my patients. Many of my patients take these popular medications at my recommendation. In my experience, there is no class of medications that people love to hate more than the statins!

One day not too long afterwards, I was seeing a patient for a regular checkup. I had recommended that the patient use a statin. He said, "Dr. Hahn, are you familiar with a radio program called *The People's Pharmacy?"* Something clicked in my brain. The conversation went something like this.

I said, "Wait a minute, did you call in to that program and talk to Dr. Sears?" His somewhat uncomfortable response was "Yes, I did."

I replied, "So when Dr. Sears said that the doctor had no idea what he was talking about, he was referring to me?"

"Yes."

Uncomfortable silence!

Friday Evening, Heart Attack;
Monday Morning, Cheeseburger

It was Friday afternoon, and if my memory serves me correctly, about 4:00 p.m. I was called to see a patient complaining of crushing chest pain and shortness of breath. He was having the classic symptoms of a heart attack. The patient was well known to me. He had a typical medical history that included all of the usual suspects: diabetes, high blood pressure, high cholesterol, and an unhealthy lifestyle.

What distinguished this patient was that we had had many conversations where I urged him to take better care of himself and he smirked and jeered at my recommendations with a classic attitude combination of "So what?" and "If I die, I die."

On this day, however, when faced with the very real possibility that he might be dying from a heart attack, the bravado melted away. Now it was: "I'm scared" and "You've gotta help me, doc!"

And help we did. But not without reminding the patient how he didn't seem so brave all of a sudden and, of course, hoping that this experience would serve as the inspiration to a change in lifestyle. We shipped the patient, via ambulance, to our local hospital, where he was quickly and appropriately assessed and then shipped, again quickly, to a big city hospital, where he promptly received a stent to the coronary artery that had been blocked. Life saved!

The most important point of this story is the miracle that is modern cardiac care. This patient came right in after developing chest pain, and we were able to fix him, preventing death, of course, but also preventing both the short- and long-term harm that used to define a heart attack.

In the old days (the 1980s and early 1990s), had this patient lived, he would have faced a future of progressively worsening heart function (congestive heart failure) that would have gradually disabled and then killed him over the next few years.

But with modern care, this patient's heart was instantly fixed; because blood flow to the heart's muscles was restored and he was prescribed a combination of important medications, it was actually likely better than it had been in years.

I spoke to the patient on Saturday morning, and he was feeling completely better, as if nothing had happened the day before. He was released from the hospital on Sunday and back in my office for a recheck on Monday.

The patient then bragged, "Hey doc, guess where I ate on the way home from the hospital?"

Yes, ladies and gentlemen, he went right back to his favorite fast-food hangout and treated his new heart to a load of the same garbage that had caused the problem in the first place!

Grrrrrrr!

Friday Night Atrial Fibrillation

I have a favorite story about diagnosing atrial fibrillation, a common type of heart rhythm abnormality where the heartbeat becomes irregular and, often, too fast.

It was a Friday night. I received a call from Maureen.

I will digress for a moment and tell a quick but unrelated story about her. When I was in medical school, I read a great book about the famed Dr. Patch Adams. The book had any number of stories and quotes that moved me so much that I kept the book on my office bookshelf and pulled it out from time to time when I needed inspiration.

I was seeing Maureen in the office one day, and she informed me that she was a writer, and that she had actually written a book about the great doctor Patch Adams. I left the exam room, went directly to my office, and pulled my Patch Adams book off the shelf. Sure enough, Maureen was the author!

Now I'll get back to the atrial fibrillation story.

Maureen stated (over the phone) that she had a funny feeling in her chest, and that her pulse was irregular. Maureen lived way out in the country and wanted to know if she needed to go to the hospital.

I asked her to feel her pulse and describe what she felt. She replied something along the lines of "Boop-boop-boop . . . boop . . . boop . . . boop-boop . . . boop . . . boop-boop-boop-boop." She was describing quite perfectly the irregular heartbeat of atrial fibrillation.

I advised Maureen to go to the hospital, where her diagnosis was confirmed.

Wonder Why My Nurse Can't Get a Pulse?

One day during my third year of residency, I was seeing patients in our residency clinic, and the nurse told me that they were bringing in a new patient who wasn't feeling well. He hadn't been to a doctor in years and just hadn't been feeling very well the last couple of weeks.

The nurse came out of the exam room and said, "Dr. Hahn, could you check this patient's pulse and blood pressure? I just can't feel the pulse, and I couldn't get a blood pressure." I went into the exam room and introduced myself. The patient seemed comfortable. I checked his pulse, but I couldn't feel anything either. I also tried to get his blood pressure, but I couldn't get a reading either. I asked the nurse to check an electrocardiogram (EKG).

A few minutes later, she handed me the EKG, and what I saw shocked me. The patient was in ventricular fibrillation (a very dangerous rapid, irregular heart rhythm), which didn't seem possible, because ventricular fibrillation is the most ominous heart rhythm abnormality, and patients with ventricular fibrillation are usually unconscious. This patient had walked into our office and did not appear to be on the way out quite yet. I went immediately to show my attending physician, who agreed with my reading.

Just as an aside, we were in a clinic that was a long hallway and one flight up from the hospital's highly regarded ER.

My attending's suggestion kind of shocked me. "Call 911," he said. "But we're in a clinic attached to the hospital," I said. "The best and safest way to get him to the ER is to call 911," he reiterated. So, feeling a bit odd, I called 911.

The squad showed up a few minutes later, got the patient on a gurney, and started an IV. Just then, he passed out and became unresponsive! I began chest compressions while EMS staff bagged him (administered breaths through a bag and mask), and medications were started through the IV. We traveled through the clinic, down the hallway, and onto the elevator, went one floor down, and then into the ER. I was doing chest compressions on the rolling gurney.

I was glad to hand the case over to the ER staff, who were much more experienced with such circumstances. The patient lived. My hair began to turn gray.

Chapter 9

Lungs/Breathing

Cough
Threat Level–Cough: LOW

Coughing, like all other symptoms that involve the lungs, may be the sign of a minor condition, such as a cold virus, that does not require medical attention or of a serious condition, such as a severe infection or even lung cancer. Coughing should receive prompt medical attention under the following circumstances:

- Cough associated with difficulty breathing
- Cough associated with a high fever
- Cough associated with weight loss
- Cough associated with significant tiredness or weakness
- Cough that produces a significant amount of blood (more than a tiny spot)

Coughing that is not associated with any of the above-mentioned conditions should receive medical attention if it does not begin to improve within 3 to 4 weeks.

Gradual Onset of Difficulty Breathing
Threat Level–Gradual onset of difficulty breathing: LOW-MEDIUM

A gradual onset of shortness of breath or difficulty breathing (gradual means symptoms that are noticed over a period of a few hours to days/

weeks/months), while not necessarily an emergency, may be a sign of a serious condition. Therefore, gradual onset shortness of breath should be checked by a doctor.

Lots of medical conditions, some that involve the lungs, such as asthma or emphysema, and even conditions that don't involve the lungs, such as anemia or heart disease, can present with the symptom of difficulty breathing. So how soon do you need to see a doctor for gradual onset of difficulty breathing? Rules to help you decide how soon you should receive medical attention:

- Severe shortness of breath, even gradual in onset, is an emergency. Seek immediate care.
- Shortness of breath that is associated with pain in the chest or that is triggered by physical exertion or stress may be a sign of heart disease. If you do not have a known medical condition, such as asthma or emphysema, you should seek immediate care.
- Mild shortness of breath not associated with chest pain or physical exertion: Gradual onset of shortness of breath that is mild in intensity should receive medical attention within 1 to 4 weeks. The severity of the shortness of breath and how quickly it is becoming worse should guide your decision about how quickly to see a doctor.

Sudden Onset of Difficulty Breathing
Threat Level—Sudden onset of difficulty breathing: VERY HIGH–HIGHEST

Let's get this on the table right away. Sudden onset of significant shortness of breath ("sudden" means symptoms begin over a period of seconds to a few hours) or difficulty breathing is an emergency of the highest order!

The lungs play an especially important role in human physiology, and without functioning lungs, it is relatively difficult to stay alive! Emergency conditions such as a blood clot in the lungs (pulmonary embolism) or a collapsed lung (pneumothorax) announce themselves with a sudden onset of shortness of breath.

To make matters worse, difficulty breathing may also be an indication of serious trouble with the heart—and the heart is also a relatively important organ. Therefore, knowing when to get medical attention for a serious lung disorder is important. Fortunately, emergency medical problems that involve the lungs are not terribly subtle. They announce themselves loud and clear.

Sudden onset of significant shortness of breath or difficulty breathing—unless you have a known lung condition, such as asthma or emphysema and know how to treat those conditions during an attack—should be treated as an emergency and should receive immediate medical attention.

Sudden Onset of Difficulty Breathing in People with Chronic Lung Conditions
Threat Level—Sudden onset of difficulty breathing with chronic lung conditions: VERY HIGH–HIGHEST

People with asthma or emphysema (or other known chronic lung condition) should seek immediate medical attention if:

- They are having severe symptoms that do not improve after one to two treatments with albuterol (or other acute breathing treatments).
- They are beginning to tire from their symptoms.

Please, Please Tell the Doctor When You're Short of Breath
This is the first part of a really good story. Part two is in the section on back pain. This first part of the story tells the tale of a classic presentation of a pulmonary embolism, a blood clot in the lungs, that took some very interesting and harrowing twists and turns.

Our story focuses on a very nice older woman (who would later sue me but, oddly, still seemed nice). She had severe chronic low back issues that eventually led to surgery, performed in Baltimore. Prior to the surgery, she was in pain and had difficulty walking because of leg weakness that related to the issues in her low back.

Following the surgery, our friend remained in the hospital for days, recovering nicely. She was anxious to get home, however. So anxious that she failed to mention to her doctors there that she had begun to feel short of breath on the day she was to be discharged. Home she went.

By the time she arrived home, about 50 miles from Baltimore, she was having a good deal of difficulty breathing. She contacted her family doctor, who also happened to be a friend, and he made a house call to check her out. That's right, he did a house call! Some of us still do that.

He confirmed that she was indeed having difficulty breathing and told her to go to her local hospital's ER. I was in training at this particular hospital, in my third year of residency. Her doctor was concerned she could have a blood clot in her lung. In fact, she had blood clots in both lungs. Blood clots are, unfortunately, more common following surgery and any period of prolonged immobilization. The next morning, I came on duty and heard about our friend, who became my patient.

The point of the story, up to this point, is that you should immediately tell your doctor if you experience a sudden onset of shortness of breath. You should especially tell your doctor this if you are in the hospital, and even more especially if you are in the hospital following surgery!

Why is it so important to tell your doctor this? Number one, because a pulmonary embolism is one of the most serious postsurgical complications that can occur. It can kill you! In this case, it did not. Number two is that, in this case, had she told her doctors in Baltimore that she was short of breath, I would not have gotten sued!

For part two of this story—which I think is more interesting—see the section on back pain.

Being There for Cookies and Soda

Ralph was in his nineties, and he was not a regular at the doctor's office. Compared to his wife, Adele, who came to see me quite often, Ralph was a veritable mystery man. So I knew it must be serious when Ralph came in complaining of a cough. I remember him also telling me that his throat felt like it was on fire way deep down. I ordered a chest x-ray, which unfortunately revealed that Ralph had lung cancer.

I called Ralph and told him that I would be dropping by the house to talk to him. Ralph was outside to greet me when I got to the house. I'll never forget what he said—"You must not be aware, Doctor, but you guys don't make house calls anymore."

I explained that when I have something serious to discuss with my patients, I prefer to do it face to face. What I didn't say was that at his age he had earned the right to get a home visit, especially under the circumstances. That's how I felt then, and I still do today.

Ralph sensed the seriousness of my mood and said, "You are aware, Doctor, that sometimes bad things happen to people my age?" That gave me a laugh. Ralph invited me in and offered me a seat in their beautifully decorated living room. Adele came in with a plate of Chips Ahoy! cookies and cans of Coca-Cola.

Before we could begin our discussion, they insisted I have a cookie and some Coke. In fact, throughout our conversation about Ralph's cancer, both Ralph and Adele seemed more concerned that I get my fill of cookies and soda than with the cancer. It felt more like a visit to my grandparents' than a doctor's appointment.

That's how house calls often go. Being in a patient's home allows for more personal interactions because the patient is on their own turf, more comfortable and more in control of their surroundings than when they are in the doctor's office.

Why do I do house calls? The simple answer is that when I was in training, a number of my favorite faculty members did them, and told me I should do them, as well. I didn't know any better, so I listened and did them. It just stuck.

One such faculty member was Dr. Stanley Talpers. The year I began medical school at George Washington University School of Medicine was the first year of a new course called "The Practice of Medicine." In that course, small groups of medical students were paired with physicians from the community. Dr. Talpers was one of the physicians who led our group. We spent a good deal of time with him, practicing such things as how to interview and examine patients. It was time well spent.

Dr. Talpers was the perfect image of the sage physician. He was tall, wore wire-rimmed glasses, and had white hair. His lab coat was always crisp, and his bearing was calm, kind, and reassuring.

One of the questions that most concerned the students in our group was what to say during difficult situations. For instance, if someone was seriously ill or dying, or even if someone had died, would we know what to say? We were terrified we would say something inappropriate.

Dr. Talpers had the answer, but what he said was surprising. He told us, in fact, that he felt the same way. But it didn't matter. What mattered far more was that we were there. He told us that, in all likelihood, no matter what we said, what patients and their families would carry forward was that we were there with them in their time of need.

"Be there," he said. It was the single best piece of advice that any of my faculty members or medical mentors gave me during my training.

That's why I do house calls—to be there. Plus, you might get cookies.

Chapter 10

The Back (Back Pain)

Back Pain
Threat Level—Back pain: LOW–MEDIUM

Here's the thing about back pain. People are always having back pain. We see a few cases of back pain every week, at least. But the *huge majority* of back pain cases are not medically important beyond the need to alleviate the pain. Granted, you may be in exquisite pain, but still, a *great majority* of the time your pain does not represent a more serious underlying medical problem.

But there is one back-pain-related emergency you must know about (the cauda equina syndrome), and there are other rare instances when back pain signals an important medical condition.

It's important to remember that, when you have pain in a bone, joint, or muscle, it is usually a minor problem, but you also have to be aware of the possibility that the pain might be a sign of three important problems:

- Broken bone
- Infection
- Cancer

In this section, we will discuss how to tell whether the pain in your back requires medical care and how quickly you need to see the doctor.

Back Pain Red Flags

Fortunately, true back pain emergencies are quite rare. For the great majority of cases, the trick is to determine whether the pain might represent a more serious underlying issue. Another way to look at this problem is that we doctors are trying to decide who needs an MRI.

MRIs are performed way too often and way too early in most cases of back pain. Doctors are taught that most people who have low back pain don't need an MRI unless the pain continues for 4 to 6 weeks. In my experience, most patients come to the doctor for pain if it has lasted 2 to 3 days. The back pain red flags are a series of alerts that doctors are taught to help them identify who needs an early MRI. Other than those who have signs of the cauda equina syndrome discussed below, people who are having back pain should contact the doctor under the following circumstances:

- Age over 50 or under 18 and no known reason for back pain
- History of cancer that has spread to the bone
- Severe pain and fever
- Significant unexplained weight loss
- Significant recent trauma or injury
- Recent spinal surgery
- Pain that lasts longer than 4 to 6 weeks

Cauda Equina Syndrome

Threat Level—Cauda equine syndrome: VERY HIGH–HIGHEST

The cauda equina syndrome is a true emergency. Think of it like a stroke that takes place in the lower back. In the cauda equine syndrome (named after the lower portion of the spinal cord, which has a shape similar to a horse's tail—*cauda* means "tail"; *equina* means "horse"), the nerves in the low back are severely compressed (by a bulging disc, swelling from blood or infection, etc.). If the nerve compression is not relieved quickly, permanent damage may occur. The symptoms of cauda equina syndrome include pain in the low back plus:

- Pain in one or both legs, often in the buttocks and traveling down the back of the legs
- Inability to control the bowels or bladder, resulting in either an inability to move the bowels or urinate, or urinary or bowel incontinence
- Weakness or numbness of the legs
- Numbness in the groin and buttocks (saddle bag anesthesia)

How quickly the cauda equine syndrome needs to be fixed is controversial, but I was taught that the sooner the better, and that patients who were treated within 6 to 12 hours had a better chance of recovery without permanent paralysis taking place.

That is why the cauda equina syndrome is a true emergency!

Why I Will Never Forget the Cauda Equina Syndrome (and Now You Won't Either)

I shared part one of this story in the "Lungs" chapter. As promised, here's the rest of the story.

A team of physicians (I was a resident physician on the team) was treating a woman with a postoperative blood clot in her lungs, a pulmonary embolism. She had undergone lower back surgery at a large university surgical center and, upon her discharge from that hospital, had become short of breath. She came to our hospital and was diagnosed with blood clots in both lungs. Appropriately, she was placed on blood thinners to help prevent further clotting.

After she had been in the hospital a few days, she began to complain of increasing pain in her low back. Chronic back pain had been the reason for her operation. One of my very astute attending physicians suggested that the patient might be bleeding into her surgical site and that the blood could be placing pressure on the nerves of the low back, causing the pain. She also had weakness of the legs, but it was difficult to know if this was an entirely new symptom because she had had weakness prior to her surgery.

The very difficult question was what to do about the blood thinners, which increase a person's risk of bleeding. On the one hand, the patient had suffered one of the most feared and dangerous postoperative complications, a blood clot. And she had blood clots in both lungs, adding to the very serious nature of her condition. In other words, blood thinners were keeping her alive.

On the other hand, she could be bleeding into her low back surgical site, causing a cauda equina syndrome. If that was the case, what should we do about the blood thinners? We asked a back specialist, an orthopedic surgeon, to consult on the case and we obtained a CAT scan of the low back to look for bleeding; at that time, our hospital did not have an MRI machine on site. The CAT scan was inconclusive.

We needed an MRI to settle the question, but we did not feel comfortable shipping such an unstable patient to the MRI facility. We did it anyway. The MRI report described a possible hemorrhage in the low back, which is what we feared.

We were in a perfect catch-22 situation. If we stopped the blood thinner, she could have another, even more tragic, blood clot. If we continued the blood thinner, she could suffer the most serious back-related condition, the cauda equina syndrome, and risked permanent nerve damage.

We decided to ship the patient back to the original surgeon. We did so with great haste, of course. This entire scenario had played out over a day or two. I felt then—and I still feel today—that a team of very talented physicians (not me, I was just a young doc, medically wet behind the ears) did as good a job as could be done under the difficult circumstances that we faced.

Two years later, I was out of residency, a practicing physician, and I received a large, thick envelope from the hospital where I had trained. Within the envelope were legal documents outlining the malpractice case that had been filed against me and the entire team of physicians who had been involved in this case.

It was not until many years later (I think it was seven) that the case actually went to trial. Two weeks prior to the beginning of the trial, I was removed as a defendant. I'm not sure why that was, but I was still called on to testify.

The medical case, as we understood it, hinged on whether we had responded quickly enough once the patient had begun to show signs, not just of back pain, but of a full-blown cauda equina syndrome. And get this: the crux of the case came down to two chart notes that I had written over an approximate 12-hour period in which I had detailed the patient's changing neurologic exam.

Images of those handwritten notes were projected onto the wall of the courtroom, and I was asked to read the notes to the court. Thankfully, I have remarkably good handwriting for a physician (this was noted in court!).

Fortunately, our hospital retained a really good attorney. All the defendants were found to be innocent of malpractice, and rightly so.

Let's just say, though, that I retain a special place in my heart for the cauda equina syndrome, and now you can, too.

The Challenges of Treating Pain

The gentleman was a new patient who had just moved back to the area. He reported to me that he had a long history of severe back pain and had been receiving narcotics from a family physician where he lived previously.

I told the patient that I did not typically take over a patient's pain-related care in such circumstances. The patient went so far as to get his old medical records. His story checked out. Still, I would not prescribe narcotic pain medication for him. I referred him to a pain specialist. He asked for a short-term narcotic prescription that would tide him over until he saw the pain specialist. Again, I told him no. Let's just say he was not happy about this.

A few weeks later, my nurse informed me that I had a call from the patient's father. He was very upset and angry.

The father told me that his son had overdosed on narcotics and that he was in a coma and showed signs of severe brain injury. He was not expected to recover. His father was angry that I had given his son those medicines. He had directed his son to my practice because he had heard that I rarely prescribed narcotics.

I was confused. My memory of the case was that I had not prescribed pain medication for his son. The few moments it took me to pull up the patient's record on the computer were agonizing.

My memory was accurate. I had not written the patient a prescription. But he had gotten a prescription at the pain management office.

As this story illustrates, taking care of pain can be complicated and challenging. Options for treating pain are often suboptimal. And I do not have a crystal ball to tell me which patients are being untruthful about their pain or are using their medications improperly. As America struggles to find ways to undo its epidemic of narcotic abuse and overuse, it would do well to avoid simplistic solutions that ignore such facts.

Chapter 11

Abdomen

Abdominal Pain

Threat Level–Abdominal pain: DEPENDS ON CIRCUMSTANCES LISTED BELOW
Threat Level–Severe abdominal pain: VERY HIGH

The abdomen usually announces that it has a problem by hurting. While other parts of the body let you know there is a problem in all sorts of ways, the abdomen is usually pretty straightforward. It speaks in the universal language of pain.

And when it comes to pain of the abdominal area, there are some relatively easy, clear-cut ways to decide who needs to see the doctor and how quickly.

Why is it important to receive care promptly for a serious cause of abdominal pain? Because prompt treatment may make a difference in who lives and who dies. For instance, if you remove the appendix quickly from someone who has appendicitis, things usually go well. If you wait too long, a burst appendix and a severe infection may be the result.

First, a quick course on deciding what is wrong. Diagnosing the cause of abdominal pain usually begins with abdominal geography. Doctors are taught to divide the abdomen into a number of anatomical sections, and the cause of the abdominal pain depends on what organs lie underneath the section where the pain is.

For simplicity, assume that pain in any area of the abdomen might be a sign of cancer (I know, this section seemed lighthearted until I wrote that). Common causes of abdominal pain by section (see Image 3):

- Upper abdomen, middle: ulcer, pancreatitis (inflammation of the pancreas), gastritis
- Upper abdomen, right side: gallstones, hepatitis (inflammation of the liver)
- Upper abdomen, left side: frankly, not much happens here
- Lower abdomen, right side: appendicitis
- Lower abdomen, left side: diverticulitis (an inflammatory condition of the bowel)
- Lower abdomen, middle: urinary infection, infections of the lady parts

Once you are thinking about the location of the pain and what organs might be affected, these general rules of thumb can guide you further:

- Sudden onset of severe abdominal pain that does not stop quickly (a minute or two) is an emergency until proven otherwise.
- The more intense the pain and the longer it lasts, the more quickly you should seek medical care.
- Any abdominal pain that does not go away quickly (1 to 5 days) and is associated with any of the following symptoms should receive prompt attention:
  - Fever
  - Weight loss
  - Blood in the stool
  - Blood in the urine
  - A noticeable growth or swelling in the abdomen
  - Change in the pattern of your bowel movements, such as constipation or diarrhea
- Any abdominal pain of unknown cause, even pain of gradual onset and mild intensity, should be evaluated by a doctor if it continues for 3 to 4 weeks.

Hernia
Threat Level—Hernia: LOW

The most common types of hernias occur when the bowel pokes through an opening in the abdominal wall, resulting in a lump or a bulge. The most common locations are around the belly button (umbilical hernia) and in the groin (inguinal hernia). Hernias are rarely a cause for alarm. If they are not painful or the cause of any other symptoms, they may not require treatment at all. Rarely, a hernia can become strangulated (cut off from its blood supply) or cause a bowel obstruction. Significant pain, redness or other discoloration, nausea, vomiting, or fever associated with a hernia are reasons to seek immediate medical care.

Indigestion
Threat Level—Indigestion: LOW-MEDIUM

Indigestion, referred to in medical circles as dyspepsia, is a catch-all term that represents various symptoms that can include nausea, heartburn, excessive gassiness, abnormal abdominal fullness, and pain. Typical causes include gastroesophageal reflux (GERD) and gastritis (irritation of the lining of the stomach), but in rare instances, indigestion can be a sign of cancer. Therefore, new-onset indigestion should be checked by a doctor within 3 to 4 weeks, or sooner if symptoms are severe.

Hahn Syndrome

Sure, now you expect that I'll tell the tale of some harrowing but educational case of abdominal pain. We'll get to that in a moment. But first I have something far more important to discuss.

It is here, in these pages, that I formally request that the medical establishment name an abdominal pain syndrome after me: *Hahn syndrome.*

Hahn syndrome would be used to describe pain of the abdomen that originates from the subcutaneous fat (the fat located just under the skin) overlying the abdomen. In other words, Hahn syndrome is pain in the belly fat!

I'm not kidding! My nurse and I can attest to this. I am the world's leading expert on this syndrome.

The year was 1999. I was a second-year family medicine resident. Unlike some resident physicians, who relax after they graduate medical school, I began to study harder in residency than I had in medical school. I studied harder because I was terrified. I had just gotten my medical degree, which meant that people were calling me "Doctor." Funny thing is, when they address you that way, they also expect that you actually know something about medicine. I didn't want to disappoint them, or kill them for that matter. So I studied and studied.

I read an article about the evaluation of abdominal pain. It was organized in the typical way, categorizing different diagnoses according to the location of the pain (as I do above). Each category had a long list of possible diagnoses. At the end of one of the lists was "Abdominal wall pain." In the text of the article was the advice to always pinch the abdominal wall fat, just in case the pain originated there. I had not heard that before. I was intrigued.

Often, after something in a medical journal catches my eye, within a few days I see a patient with that very same problem.

And so it was that one day, shortly after reading this article about abdominal pain, that a young lady came to see me—with abdominal pain. Her story was similar to one that I would hear many times over the ensuing years. She had been having pain of the abdomen for months, sometimes quite severe pain. All her testing—the labs, the scans—was normal. The concern for her was so great (because her pain was so severe) that she had just had exploratory surgery to find the source of the pain. The surgeon found nothing! She was quite uncomfortable on that fateful day that the gods of medicine sent her my way.

As I heard her story, I worried, "How will I be able to figure out the cause of her pain when so many (probably far more experienced) doctors had failed before me?"

As I examined her abdomen, I visualized the underlying body parts. She writhed and groaned when I examined her lower abdomen. But all the testing, and then the surgery, would have isolated the cause of her pain. I wracked my brains. I remembered then to pinch the abdominal wall fat overlying the area of her pain.

She screamed! I pinched again, this time apologizing for pinching her—again she screamed. I did something interesting after that. I filled a syringe with lidocaine, a numbing medicine, and injected the lidocaine under the skin where my pinches had elicited such pain (I think this was actually suggested in the article I had read. But sometimes when I tell this story and I'm really in the mood to embellish, I take credit for this idea).

Her pain went away! She was pain free for the first time in months. I was as surprised as she was, but in proper doctor fashion, I hid this fact from her. I assured her that she would be better from then on. I scheduled her to return back one month later.

The next appointment, she told me that her pain had left entirely for a couple of weeks, but then returned, though it was far less severe than before. I decided to inject the lidocaine again. Her pain was gone for good!

I realize that there must be some other doctor who knows about abdominal wall fat pain syndrome (at least the author of that article I had read), but I have yet to meet another doctor who can diagnose this. Nor have I read about it in any other article, and I have read many thousands of articles since then.

Soon after treating this sentinel case of what I would later refer to as *Hahn syndrome*, a similar case presented to me. Again I injected lidocaine. Again the pain resolved, and then again, and again, and again.

What is so striking to me is that so often the patient has already seen a number of doctors and has had all the proper testing, but no one was able to tell them that they had pain of the abdominal wall fat. As the years progressed, I recognized that abdominal wall fat pain tends to be localized most often to the right upper quadrant, just beneath the rib cage. It also can occur in the fat of the lowest portions of the abdomen, on the right or the left, but it is most frequent in the right uppermost abdomen.

I have helped many people over the years get over the pain of Hahn syndrome!

Is It Appendicitis or Not?

One of the classic, most iconic, and important causes of abdominal pain is appendicitis. Most people know that one cause of severe abdominal pain is appendicitis, and many also know the location of the appendix, which is typically found in the lower right portion of the abdomen.

On this last point, though, I am reminded of an episode of the great TV comedy *Scrubs*. JD was admitted to the hospital with abdominal pain. The next morning, the medical team was rounding and came to his bedside. The doctor pressed on the *left side* (the wrong side) of his abdomen and diagnosed appendicitis. Off to surgery he went. I loved that show.

Of course, as a doctor, I know it is extremely important to diagnose appendicitis in a timely fashion. An appendectomy early in the course of appendicitis is a relatively minor procedure. Wait too long and you risk a burst appendix, which can be a mess for both the patient and the surgeon.

But what fun would medicine be if proper diagnosis of appendicitis were always easy? I assure you, it is not (at least, it isn't always). Some patients with appendicitis look horribly uncomfortable—these are the easy cases—but some look just fine. Some patients are so tender they jump when you press on their abdomen, but some aren't tender at all. To make matters worse, diagnostic testing such as a CAT scan is very good but not perfect.

Throw into the mix the fact that insurance companies and hospitals are pressuring doctors to order fewer tests, so the doctor has to think not just about what is best for the patient, but also what is most profitable for the hospital and insurance company. This makes for real drama.

The classic presentation of appendicitis is pain of the lower abdomen, most often in the lower right abdomen, though sometimes at the beginning, the pain is a little over to the left. The pain usually progresses to be rather severe over a relatively brief amount of time, a few hours to 1 or 2 days max.

One of the first cases I was to encounter during residency was a patient who came in to our ER one evening. He had developed right lower abdominal pain earlier in the day, which had been fairly severe at first, but decreased quite a bit by the time I met him. I examined the patient, and there was no tenderness at all. He couldn't have looked more comfortable.

I presented the case to my ER attending, one of the more experienced doctors with whom we worked. He wanted to know what I thought, of course, and what I thought was that the patient couldn't have appendicitis because he looked fine and had no tenderness when I examined him.

My attending did something that I will always remember. He told me to send the patient home but have him return early in the morning. When the patient returned, the doctor said, he would have full-blown appendicitis, and we would send him to surgery. This was an interesting approach. Sure enough, when the patient returned, he was again experiencing pain, and now he was tender in the right spot. Off to surgery he went.

So there were two things that interested me about that early case. First was the fact that this patient's pain came and went and then came back in the way that it did. I had been under the impression that someone with appendicitis would develop pain that would be unrelenting and would predictably worsen with time. Obviously, this was not always the case.

Second was the combination of intuition and experience my attending physician utilized to make the correct diagnosis. This seemed as much stylish art as science to me. It was one of the moments that would help me to fall in love with my profession, to help give me the sense that I had a calling, not just a job. I began to understand the phrase "the art of medicine."

A year or so later, I was a newly minted practicing physician, working in a small town in rural western Maryland at a community health center. In an odd turn of events, I had also been asked to be the center's medical director, despite the fact that I was the new kid on the block. I saw this for what it probably was: a bit of an honor, but also a sign that something must be wrong.

Soon after I began, one of my colleagues, a physician assistant, far more experienced than I was at that point, consulted me for my opinion about a patient who had been experiencing right lower abdominal pain. I went to the exam room, where I found the patient appearing to be completely comfortable. The patient had begun to have pain overnight, and it had been significantly painful initially but eased up quite a bit by the time I saw him. On exam, there was minimal tenderness when I pressed deeply over the painful area.

As much as I wanted to make the correct diagnosis for the sake of the patient, I also knew that the eyes of the staff were upon me and that I had a chance to let them know what their new colleague was made of. I would characterize their attitude toward me at that time as somewhere between passive-aggressive (hoping I would fail) and open hostility (I was a newcomer, an outsider, and had been placed in charge of far more experienced staff).

My assessment was that appendicitis was unlikely. The patient appeared too well, was experiencing very mild symptoms, and had an unimpressive exam. Before discharging the patient, I gave the warning, as I was taught to do, that he should call us or go to the ER if the pain returned.

My assessment turned out to be wrong. The patient had surgery that night. Fortunately, it was a "no harm, no foul" situation. The surgery went well, and the patient did well. Lesson learned, also.

The next challenging case turned out to be that of my daughter. Willa was seven or eight years old at the time and, much to her chagrin, was at a week-long sleepover camp—where there was no TV. We received a call to report that our darling was complaining of right lower abdomen pain.

Growing up, Willa was very active in our local community theater and had developed quite the dramatic flair. She also heard tales every night of my most interesting and challenging cases, and I think she wanted to get in on the action. Of course, the stakes can't get much higher than when a physician is considering the health of his own child. On the one hand, Willa looked fine and had an unrevealing physical exam. I did not want to overreact. On the other hand, I didn't want to be the foolish physician (and father) who missed appendicitis in his own daughter, for a number of obvious reasons. My thinking was "better safe than sorry," which is rarely a bad philosophy when it comes to health-care decision making.

The hospital was about 30 miles to the south. The physician who evaluated Willa—who by that time was smiling and clearly enjoying our little adventure—was kind and understanding. She ordered a CAT scan, which was normal. Willa was fine. We went home. She stayed fine. She got to watch TV.

Sometime after that, I finally saw a classic case of appendicitis. An elderly patient came into the office, bent over from pain, holding her right side. She grunted and writhed when I pressed on her abdomen. Off to the hospital she went, where the diagnosis was confirmed and successful surgery performed.

Since then, I have seen numerous cases of appendicitis. I have evaluated a number of patients with right lower abdominal pain who turn out not to have appendicitis; there are other causes of pain in that area. I have not missed a diagnosis since that early case mentioned above.

There was the time, just a couple of years ago, when we received a call from a mom whose young son was seen the day before at the local hospital for abdominal pain. I knew Mom as the bartender at our small town's most wonderful restaurant—not someone you want to disappoint!

They were told at the hospital that it was just a stomach bug. Her son failed to improve, though, and, in fact, he had spent the ensuing night writhing on the floor because of his pain. She was calling for advice. We had never seen her son as a patient. We brought him right in. He was indeed tender in the right lower abdomen. We sent him directly to another hospital, where he was operated on for his appendicitis.

Well, medicine has a great way, just when you're beginning to feel good about your skills (and not losing sleep worrying about them), of reminding you that you are fallible. About a year ago, a patient came in with the perfect story for appendicitis. The pain had begun overnight, he appeared uncomfortable, and he was quite tender in just the right place when I examined him. It was a no-brainer. I sent him to the ER for evaluation.

I received a call from the ER physician who wanted to let me know that the CAT scan showed a case of "epiploic appendagitis" and the patient was being sent home with some anti-inflammatory medications.

I said, "What did you say?" Again I got the answer, "epiploic appendagitis." I looked this up on the computer in front of me, and there it was. As Wikipedia informed me, "epiploic appendagitis is an uncommon, benign, non-surgical, self-limiting inflammatory process of the . . . small, fat-filled sacs along the surface of the upper and lower colon."

OK, there I was, a practicing physician for many years, and I had not heard this diagnosis before? The ER doc said, "Yeah, we see about a case every year." I was embarrassed and a little upset. I called my good doctor buddy, Shawn Moyer, also a practicing family physician, and asked him if he were aware of this diagnosis. Thankfully, he was not. I was not alone! Dr. Moyer asked his wife, who is also a physician, a very experienced practicing internist, if she had heard of epiploic appendagitis. She had not, either! I was comforted.

For good measure, Dr. Moyer proceeded to tell me an appendicitis story of his own. One day, two family members had been brought to his office, both complaining of the same stomach bug. A virus had been going around their community. The first patient checked out fine. It was most likely the same stomach bug many other community members were experiencing. The fact that two members of the same family had similar symptoms made the diagnosis much more likely, of course. Dr. Moyer was tempted not to even examine the second family member, who had the same symptoms, over the same time period, and almost assuredly had the same diagnosis. A diligent doctor, though, Dr. Moyer performed the exam. The second patient had appendicitis!

Not as easy as it seems, eh?

Grace

Glenn was one of my favorite patients. He died years ago, but I keep his picture on my exam room desk.

Glenn was the father of one of my best nurses, and he was the well-known owner of a popular local hunting and sporting goods store. I also took care of a number of Glenn's family members and countless friends and acquaintances. We always had a great time during Glenn's appointments. He was a great teller of tales, especially about his outdoor experiences. He liked to give me advice about fly-fishing. I was a novice fly-fisher at the time. Of note, Glenn taught me his tried-and-true method for removing a hook from a fish's mouth.

It was particularly painful when one summer Glenn began to have abdominal pain and we diagnosed him with pancreatic cancer. It is still painful to think about. Typical of Glenn, though, he took the news with remarkable grace.

As many people know, pancreatic cancer is one of the most serious cancers. It is often too late to treat pancreatic cancer when a patient develops symptoms and is diagnosed. Unfortunately, that was the case with Glenn.

Glenn's number one concern was his family. It is an understatement to say that Glenn was revered by his family. Notably, every fall Glenn took select family members along on a hunting trip out west. It was a chance to get away from the business, but also to spend special time with loved ones. Glenn wanted to make sure he could still go. I don't think it mattered what I told him, though. He was going on that trip!

Glenn must have suffered greatly on that trip. He came to see me very soon after returning. His legs were swollen, and he was having a good deal of difficulty breathing. He had developed blood clots in his lungs. It was hard to keep up with the number of complications that Glenn developed because of his cancer. One of the problems in treating him was that he would never complain despite what must have been horrific suffering.

By the Christmas and New Year's holidays, things had progressed to the point that I felt it was time to discuss hospice care. I went to Glenn's home on New Year's Day for the conversation. I brought my young daughter along because I wanted her to meet Glenn, to witness such grace in the face of such difficult circumstances.

I sat with Glenn in his den. He recollected how his family's first home had burned down and how he had rebuilt the house himself, collecting by hand many large stones from his land that now adorned the walls and fireplace where we sat.

Hanging all around the room were fiddles. There were twenty to thirty, if memory serves me correctly. Glenn had made every one of them. They each had a tag on them with a person's name on it. Glenn told me that each one was going to a friend or family member who he thought would enjoy it.

It was a difficult end-of-life conversation. At one point, Glenn interrupted me, "Dr. Hahn, you seem upset. Are you OK?" So, in Glenn's time of greatest need, it was he who was comforting me, his physician. That was Glenn.

Glenn's daughter, Debbie, told me that Glenn spent time with each and every family member, making sure that they had what they needed, that they each knew how special they were to him; he also tried to advise them going forward in their lives. He passed away nineteen days later, surrounded by his family.

About a month later, I was seeing patients when I was informed that Debbie and Mabel, Glenn's wife, had come to the office and wanted to see me. I didn't know why they had come. I was actually afraid that they might be angry with me.

On the contrary, they had a gift for me. It was one of Glenn's fly rods. It came with a reel that had an automatic line-retrieve button. I had never seen one before. They felt that Glenn would have wanted me to have the rod and reel. It was an incredible honor. I went to Yellowstone National Park later that year, to the Yellowstone River, where Glenn liked to fish, and I fished the Yellowstone with his rod and reel.

When we opened our office in 2009, I asked Debbie for a picture of Glenn. They gave me a picture of Glenn holding that same fly rod and reel. I keep that picture on my desk for use when I have particularly difficult conversations with other patients.

I tell those patients about Glenn. He showed me that despite the most horrific circumstances, and even in death, we have the capacity, even the opportunity, to show immense grace and courage, and to maintain our dignity no matter what is happening.

Chapter 12

Urinary System (Plumbing)

Blood in the Urine
Threat Level—Blood in the urine: MEDIUM

Simple message here: visible blood in the urine is always a reason to see a doctor.

Blood in the urine has a number of well-known causes, such as a urinary infection and kidney stones. In addition, a number of common foods (certain berries, beets, food coloring) and medicines (sulfa drugs, phenazopyridine [also known as pyridium], and metronidazole) can turn the urine red or orange.

But visible blood in the urine can also be a sign of cancer, especially bladder cancer, so seeing blood in the urine should always prompt a visit to the doctor in the near future. Bladder cancer is usually quite treatable, so don't fret too much, just get to the doctor.

How soon do you need to go to a doctor?

- If you have visible blood in the urine, but no signs of urinary infection or kidney stones (see below), you should get to the doctor in the near future (1 to 2 weeks). If you feel poorly in any way, go sooner.
- If you have visible blood in the urine *and* signs of urinary infection—pain or burning with urination, difficulty urinating, more frequent urination, and possibly fever or back pain—you should go as soon as possible. Most urinary

infections are infections of the bladder, which are usually easy to treat. On the other hand, infections of the kidney, which usually have more severe symptoms, such as fever and back pain, are serious and should be treated as quickly as possible.

- A bladder infection, even though it is a relatively minor infection, if left untreated, can go on to become a kidney infection. This is the main reason a bladder infection should be treated as quickly as possible.

- If you have visible blood in the urine and *signs of a kidney stone* (usually back pain, which can be quite severe), you may need treatment for the pain. The pain of a kidney stone can be very impressive. If you have had kidney stones, or you are having one, you know what I mean. You will seek care as quickly as you can to get treatment for the pain.

- Most kidney stones will pass on their own, though some, usually the larger ones, require medical assistance to leave.

Other Urinary Symptoms

This section deals with abnormal urinary symptoms—problems with the plumbing—other than visible blood, including:

- Urinating more frequently than is usual
- Inability to urinate (or difficulty urinating)
- Pain or burning with urination
- Feeling an abnormal urge to urinate (urgency)
- Feeling the need to urinate, but having difficulty urinating (hesitance)
- Loss of bladder control (incontinence)
- Discharge from the urinary opening

Let me start with this. Where I live, it is easier to find a urologist than a plumber.

Lots of things go wrong with our plumbing. The trick is to know when a plumbing problem is a sign of a serious problem.

Most people know the signs of a urinary tract infection (UTI). The most common symptoms of a UTI include a burning feeling with urination, feeling the need to urinate more frequently, urgency, and hesitance. UTIs are quite common in women, less so in men.

A UTI can be anything from a mild annoyance to a real pain. A UTI is not usually an emergency, but it should be treated promptly because untreated, a simple UTI, which usually involves only the bladder, can move up the pipes and affect the kidneys. A kidney infection is more serious.

UTI symptoms that include fever or pain in the middle of the back may indicate a kidney infection. A kidney infection should be treated immediately.

Urinating more frequently than usual might also be a sign of diabetes; the urinary frequency wouldn't be accompanied by burning or irritation, though. The classic signs of diabetes are more frequent urination, weight loss, and abnormal thirst (all three of those might not occur, however).

But let's get down to the nitty-gritty. Use the following rules of thumb to determine when you should see a doctor for urinary symptoms:

- Urinary symptoms accompanied by fever or significant pain should be evaluated as soon as possible—within 24 hours. If your doctor can't see you, go to the ER.
- UTI symptoms without fever or significant pain should be seen promptly but are not an emergency. I would urge these people to be seen the same day, but 1 to 3 days is probably reasonable, as long as you are otherwise feeling well.
- Urinary symptoms other than a UTI, and not accompanied by fever or significant pain, should be evaluated in the near future. Usually, a few days to a couple of weeks are OK.

Oh Brother

This story is about one of the moments that inspired my writing this book.

There are certain symptoms in medicine that are so iconic that when they are heard by a trained physician, the diagnosis comes to mind instantaneously. This is a story about one of those symptoms.

One day, I received a call at the office from my brother, who was in his forties at the time. He was calling because he had seen bright red blood in his urine. I told him this was bladder cancer until proven otherwise. He needed to get it checked because it is usually quite treatable.

He got it checked. It was bladder cancer. He has been treated successfully. You should never forget this story or this lesson.

Name That Tune

It would take a whole other book to tell you all about Joltin' Jim McCoy. The very short version is that Joltin' Jim is a legendary figure in country music. He discovered the great Patsy Cline while he was a teenage performer (Jim was sixteen and Patsy was fourteen at the time) on his own live country music radio show. Jim also had a fine career as a performer (under the name Joltin' Jim McCoy and the Melody Playboys); as a well-known radio DJ in Winchester, Virginia; as a music producer; and later, as the owner of West Virginia's greatest honky-tonk bar, The Troubadour Lounge, located in the hills outside Berkeley Springs.

Joltin' Jim was a patient of mine for a few years before I found out about his musical past. We became fast friends after that, and I even recorded an album (a fine album, I might add) of Jim's songs (I had a musical past before medicine).

Anyway, not too long ago, Jim mentioned that we should record a second album of his songs. Prior to the first recording sessions, we had gone through a great deal of his music, some of which he had recorded professionally (he even had some regional hits), and some of which were just rough demos. I remembered one song in particular, a slower song that Jim and I had both really liked.

The problem was that I just couldn't remember the name of that song. I looked through old tapes, CDs, and lyric sheets that I had accumulated during the first recording sessions. I just couldn't find it. I asked Jim, and he also had a recollection of the song but couldn't remember the name either. We wracked our brains, but to no avail.

Remember, Joltin' Jim was a patient as well. He came in to the office one day with a urinary complaint. As usual, he was accompanied by his wife, Bertha.

"What's the problem, Jim? Are you having trouble urinating?" I asked. Jim drawled, "Yeah, Matt, you see, I want to, but then I can't." Something odd clicked in my brain. I am not making this up. "Wait a second, Jim, what did you just say?" I asked. Jim replied, "I said I want to, but I just can't."

"Jim!" I exclaimed. "That's the name of the song—the song we've been trying to remember is called 'Want To.'"

Chapter 13

The Bowels and Rectum (Sewer Line)

Blood: Rectal Bleeding or Blood in the Stool

Threat Level—Rectal bleeding: MEDIUM

Threat Level—Rectal bleeding and *weakness, difficulty breathing, dizziness, or pale/cool skin: VERY HIGH*

This is a tough topic, I know, but we have to deal with it. There are two major concerns related to blood from this part of the body:

- Cancer
- Bleeding emergency

Most bleeding from the bowel does *not* represent an emergency or cancer, but both possibilities need to be considered. Therefore, blood from this part of the body must be taken seriously, and it must be evaluated in a timely fashion.

The most common causes of rectal bleeding or blood in the stool are hemorrhoids and rectal fissures, diverticulosis (more about this further on), inflammatory bowel diseases, polyps in the colon, and colon cancer. Taking aspirin or NSAIDs (nonsteroidal anti-inflammatory drugs, such as ibuprofen or naproxen) on a regular basis increases the risk of bleeding.

Diverticulosis is a very common condition. Diverticulosis is the formation of small pouches in the wall of the colon. Diverticulosis can be a cause of bleeding, which can sometimes be quite serious. However, the bleeding associated with diverticulosis is usually painless, so that's a bonus.

How quickly you need to see a doctor for rectal bleeding depends on the severity of the bleeding. Heavy, continuous rectal bleeding is an emergency and requires medical attention immediately. In addition, seek immediate medical care for rectal bleeding that is associated with:

- Weakness
- Shortness of breath
- Dizziness or lightheadedness
- Pale or cool skin

Any person over the age of 40 who has rectal bleeding or blood in the stool needs to be evaluated for cancer. Mild bleeding or bleeding that is not associated with any of the symptoms listed above is not an emergency, but it should still be evaluated in the near future, within 1 to 2 weeks.

Change in Bowel Habits
Threat Level—Change in bowel habits: LOW

This is extremely important. You should be screened for colon cancer. Most people, beginning at age 50 (earlier for some, especially those whose parent or sibling had colon cancer), should get a colonoscopy or another accepted form of colon cancer screening, such as testing the stool for blood, and continue the screenings on a regular basis thereafter. If your first colonoscopy was normal and you don't have significant colon cancer risk factors, you don't have to go again for 10 years!

A change in bowel habits might include any of the following:

- Diarrhea or constipation
- Change in the size, shape, or consistency of your bowel movements

- Blood in the stool (see section above)
- Persistent abdominal pain or painful bowel movements
- Bowels not emptying completely

A persistent change in bowel habits, especially if you are older—colon cancer is more common in people over the age of 50—may be a sign of serious disease, such as cancer of the colon. Of course, most people with a change in bowel habits will not necessarily have cancer, so don't panic! Just take it seriously and see a doctor.

A persistent change in bowel habits that lasts more than a week should prompt a call to the doctor and an appointment in the near future, within 1 to 2 weeks.

My First Colonoscopy

This is a true story.

Colonoscopy is an important rite of passage for all 50-year-olds, so when my turn came, wanting to set a good example for my patients, I signed up.

My nurse, Lindy, delightedly made my referral appointment to the gastroenterologist. To do this great honor, I selected a gastroenterologist in our area who has performed the procedure on a great many of my patients, always getting rave reviews from them.

An idea occurred to me. OK, a weird idea occurred to me.

All of my patients moan and complain about their colonoscopy, especially about the dreaded bowel prep the day before. As I like to say to them, though, "It's better than colon cancer!"

This next sentence is possibly the only serious aspect of this story, so pay attention now. The fact is, I have practiced my entire career in the era of the screening colonoscopy, I recommend the procedure to every appropriate patient, and I have never had a patient who gets colonoscopies on a regular basis die from colon cancer. That makes me happy.

OK, back to our story. It is too bad that colonoscopies get such a bad rap with patients, and I hate to think of the patients who avoid the procedure because of its negative reputation.

With a tiny bit of serious intent, I hatched a plan to turn my colonoscopy into a celebration. The idea was that I would find a small group of people who all were due for their colonoscopies, transport everyone in a limo, and take them out to lunch for their post-colonoscopy meal. I would get media coverage of the "celebration," and we could show the world that a colonoscopy doesn't have to be so bad.

Initially, the plan went well. I quickly found four other people who needed the procedure, and we all got scheduled for a colonoscopy the same day, a Monday. I had contacted the limo owner, and he was available.

Unfortunately, shortly thereafter, three of the people canceled. There were only two of us left, Bill and I. Bill and I are friends, and we decided to go together anyway, both for moral support and because I needed a ride. As an added benefit, Bill is hilarious.

I needed a ride because my wife was out of town over the weekend, but she was coming home on Monday and would be driving through Hagerstown, where the procedure was taking place, so she would be able to pick us up and take us home. I purposefully scheduled my bowel prep for a Sunday when I would be alone in the house, just me and the bathroom. I just needed a way to get to Hagerstown. Bill's wife would take us there.

There I was, all alone on Sunday, as planned, as I began my bowel prep. To my surprise, I received a text from Bill, "Supposed to drink magnesium sulfate at 2:00 p.m. without alcohol. Let the fun begin." A little later, when my prep began to have its intended effect, I texted back, "Fun time is now!"

6:00 p.m., Bill: "I'm starved lol."

6:04 p.m., Me: "I have bullion, jello, and popsicles. I'm too bloated to feel hungry yet. Watching Charlie's Angels . . . dogs wait outside the bathroom each time I go. Fun."

6:10 p.m., Bill: "Rule #1 never trust a fart."

6:18 p.m., Me: "I can't believe they don't tell u about this part in more detail. Had I not known what to expect, I'd be scared as hell right now."

6:18 p.m., Me: "I'm running out of TP."

7:00 p.m., Bill: "I leave I come back I leave I oh crap I'm not leavin."

7:01 p.m., Me: "This is awesome."

7:02 p.m., Bill: "I brought my laptop into the toilet."

9:13 p.m., Bill: "Can't believe I'm still wearing pants . . . why?"

9:16 p.m., Me: "I changed into pajamas a long time ago."

9:19 p.m., Me: "I'm just going out of habit now."

This hilarity certainly helped me get through the day. As you may know, we had to repeat the whole thing in the wee hours of the morning. All in all, it wasn't so bad.

Bill came to get me in the morning. To my surprise, instead of Bill's wife driving us, it was Bill's parents. There we were, two 50-year-old men, being taken to the doctor by his mom and dad.

Even better, soon after we arrived and took our places in the waiting room, an elderly woman showed up, and she knew Bill and his parents by name. This was Bill's aunt. She was coming to wait with us, too! How sweet is that? His parents and aunt! It was touching and embarrassing at the same time.

Bill and I were called in to the preop area at about the same time. We were placed in adjacent beds. We cackled like little kids until our respective times came, and we were wheeled off to our doom.

In the OR, I was positioned for the procedure and given the great anesthetic Propofol. In what seemed like just a few minutes,

I awoke, feeling fine. They brought us excellent cookies (delicious Lorna Doones!) and soda. I had seconds. I felt fine. As you may be aware, after a colonoscopy, they want you to fart, which is fun, because usually people don't want you to do that.

My wonderful wife came in soon thereafter. But get this: Bill's mom insisted on staying until I was out of the procedure, just to make sure I was OK. Is that sweet or what? Oh yeah, my colonoscopy was completely clean. I don't get to do that again for another 10 years!

Get your colonoscopy. Don't fret too much. Go with a friend! You too can have this great a time! Remember, it's better than colon cancer.

Chapter 14

Lady Parts

Lady Parts 101: The Missed Period
Threat Level—Missed period: LOW

A missed period, or periods, might mean you're pregnant. This applies only to females. If only to save yourself the embarrassment, but for lots of even better reasons, don't be the woman who shows up at the doctor's office or ER delivering a baby when you didn't even know you were pregnant (see story below)!

If you miss a period or two and the reason isn't already apparent, check to see if you are pregnant.

Lady Parts 201: Abnormal Vaginal Bleeding, Vaginal Discharge, Pelvic Pain, Growths, or Swelling
Threat Level—Abnormal vaginal bleeding: LOW
Threat Level—Abnormal vaginal bleeding and weakness, difficulty breathing, dizziness, or pale/cool skin: VERY HIGH
Threat Level—Vaginal discharge: MEDIUM–HIGH
Threat Level—Pelvic pain, growths, or swelling: MEDIUM–HIGH

This is a catch-all section for the female reproductive organs.

Rule 1: If you are pregnant, or think you may be pregnant, and you have vaginal bleeding, vaginal discharge, or persistent or significant pelvic or lower abdominal pain, call your doctor.

Rule 2: Women aged 21 to 65 should get regular checks, including, for most women, Pap smears every 3 to 5 years to check for cervical cancer. By the way, besides receiving a Pap smear, there is no specific reason for a pelvic exam in a woman who is not having gynecologic symptoms. In other words, there is no good reason to have an annual pelvic exam.

Rule 3: Signs of infection of the female genitals—vaginal, cervical, uterine, the fallopian tubes, or the ovaries—include pelvic or lower abdominal pain, vaginal discharge, and possibly, abnormal vaginal bleeding. If you have any of these symptoms, and especially if they are accompanied by fever, nausea or vomiting, or severe pain, contact your doctor as soon as possible.

Rule 4: In women of childbearing age, irregular vaginal bleeding is extremely common, but in rare circumstances can be an indication of a serious condition. Persistent or very heavy irregular vaginal bleeding should prompt a visit to the doctor.

Rule 5: Signs of ovarian cancer can be vague and nonspecific. They may include:

- Pelvic or abdominal pain
- Abdominal bloating or swelling
- Change in appetite, feeling full more quickly, or an upset stomach
- Urinary urgency or frequency
- Change in bowel habits, such as constipation
- Pain with sex

As I said, these symptoms are relatively vague and do not necessarily indicate that you have ovarian cancer. But you and your doctor need to maintain a healthy index of suspicion when any of these symptoms occur. Symptoms that persist for 2 to 4 weeks or are severe should prompt a call to your doctor.

Postmenopausal Bleeding

Threat Level—Vaginal bleeding in a post-menopausal woman: MEDIUM
Threat Level—Vaginal bleeding and weakness, difficulty breathing, dizziness, or pale/cool skin: VERY HIGH

Any abnormal or especially heavy vaginal bleeding can be a sign of a serious medical condition. In a woman who is postmenopausal and has stopped having regular periods, vaginal bleeding should never be ignored.

Vaginal bleeding in a postmenopausal woman is uterine cancer until proven otherwise. Any vaginal bleeding in a postmenopausal woman should be evaluated by a doctor as soon as possible.

One of My Favorite Stories of All Time

All doctors hear of these legendary cases, but few get the call themselves.

Many years back, a young lady came to my office complaining of back pain. When she was scheduled by the front desk staff, I can guarantee you that the thinking was that we better get her in quickly because she might have a urinary infection. That was good thinking as far as I was concerned.

She was squeezed in for an appointment that day because it is so important to catch and treat a UTI early in its course, and this is usually a quick and easy visit. She was scheduled for just before lunchtime. I was hungry, so I was hoping for a quick appointment.

She appeared comfortable. She was maybe a little overweight. She said that she had been having low back pain that came and went in waves over the last day or so. We considered the usual causes of back pain, like a muscle strain. We checked the urine for infection, but there were none of the typical findings that indicate infection. I did a brief exam, listening to her heart and lungs and examining her back. All were normal.

She denied being sexually active. I was about to send her home with a course of antibiotics, just to be safe (thinking it might be a UTI, even though the urine was clear), but something was bothering me about this case.

Something was bothering my nurse, Lindy, as well. I was in our medicine closet, looking for an appropriate antibiotic to give her. At that moment, Lindy showed up in the medicine closet (it was a big closet) and we conferred. We were both thinking the same thing (Lindy is smarter than most doctors, so she deserves a shout out!): "Let's give her a pregnancy test."

The pregnancy test was positive. In other words, she was pregnant! Only when I saw these results did it dawn on me. Back pain that came and went . . . could she be in labor?! This was unlikely. She told me that she was not sexually active. She did not look pregnant.

I went back to speak to the patient, and to reexamine her. Her last sexual encounter, it turns out, had been about nine months earlier. Her lower abdomen was taut, and I felt what I thought was a firm, enlarged uterus, confirming my suspicions. So, not only was she pregnant, it was likely that she was in labor! Her back pains that came and went, in waves, were contractions!

She delivered that afternoon.

I love being a doctor.

The Reason I Wrote This Book

The patient was a woman who happened also to be a good friend and someone whom I admire a great deal. She came to me for a preoperative evaluation prior to a planned hysterectomy. Her gynecologist had diagnosed uterine cancer, and she needed approval for surgery that was going to be done by one of the area's gynecologic surgeons.

She was many years postmenopausal. She had gone to her gynecologist initially because she had been experiencing vaginal bleeding for the past 8 months. Vaginal bleeding in a post-menopausal woman, I knew, was uterine cancer until proven otherwise.

Eight months was a long time to have waited. As we spoke, and as I went through the presurgical evaluation, I couldn't help but worry that my friend had waited much too long, and that her cancer may have spread. Had she known the implications of postmenopausal vaginal bleeding, I'm sure she would have gone much sooner. I hoped it was not too late for her.

Fortunately, it was not. She had the surgery, and it turned out that her cancer was still in the earliest stage. The odds were extremely good that she would do well, and she did not need any follow-up chemotherapy. She was lucky. Lucky is a good thing to be.

But you shouldn't depend on it.

In the days after we got that good news, I thought long and hard about the case. It reminded me too much of the many times I have seen people who received their diagnosis too late, who were not so lucky.

This book is the result.

Chapter 15

Man Parts

Swelling of the Uncircumcised Penis: Paraphimosis
Threat Level—Paraphimosis: VERY HIGH

Paraphimosis occurs only in uncircumcised males and is a condition when the foreskin becomes trapped behind the head of the penis. Paraphimosis is an emergency because the trapped foreskin can form a band around the shaft of the penis so tight that the blood supply to the end of the penis can become cut off, resulting in gangrene.

Paraphimosis is different from another, usually less serious, issue called phimosis, where the foreskin becomes stuck in front of the head of the penis and cannot be retracted.

Symptoms of paraphimosis usually include a painful penis as well as swelling of the head of the penis.

Paraphimosis should be treated as an emergency, and you should seek medical care immediately. Paraphimosis makes me thankful for my circumcision.

Testicle Lump
Threat Level—Testicle lump: LOW-MEDIUM

A growth or lump on the testicle might be a sign of testicular cancer. Because of Lance Armstrong's experience, most men are aware of the signs of testicular cancer. Let's give Lance his due on this one. He's gotten a lot of bad press, and deservedly so, but let's remember that he did make this positive contribution, and that, despite an advanced case of testicular cancer, he was treated and cured.

The most common sign of testicular cancer is a painless lump. If you find a lump on the testicle, you should see your doctor in the near future to have it checked.

While it is important to have a lump on the testicle checked by a doctor, I would also add that normal testicles are lumpy. In fact, in my experience as a doctor, far more boys and men have come to me because they are concerned about their normal lumpy scrotums and testicles than anything else.

Most men are not familiar with the epididymis, which is a normal part of the man parts and is basically a lump on the back of the testicle. I would like to suggest right now that every man reach down and become familiar with his normal male anatomy, which will feel like a lump coming off the back side of the testicle! Now, take a moment to refocus.

Anyway, let's be clear. If you have a lump on the testicle, and especially one that is changing or growing, it should be checked by the doctor. You should also be checked for any swelling of the testicle or any persistent pain.

Testicle Pain
Threat Level—Severe testicle pain: VERY HIGH

Severe pain of the testicle or scrotum should be considered an emergency, and you should seek immediate care. While there are a number of reasons you may have pain in the testicle or scrotum, sudden severe pain may indicate what is known as torsion of the testicle. Torsion of the testicle, where the cord that attaches to the back of the testicle becomes twisted, is a true emergency because the testicle is getting cut off from its blood supply and is dying. If torsion of the testicle is not treated quickly, within hours, the testicle may die and need to be removed.

Therefore, sudden severe pain of the testicle should be treated as a true emergency, and you should go immediately to the ER.

Chapter 16

Arms and Legs

Deep Venous Thrombosis (DVT or blood clot)
Threat Level—DVT: HIGH–VERY HIGH

Aside from the obvious bad things that happen to arms and legs, such as injuries, bites, broken bones, and, of course, when arms and legs suddenly stop working (see "Stroke" in Chapter 17: Neurology), the one medical issue that affects arms and legs (but especially legs) that you need to know about is a blood clot.

Blood clots, known in medical circles as DVTs in the legs (and less frequently, in the arms) are important because they can break free and travel to the lungs, resulting in a pulmonary embolism (blood clot in the lungs), which can be severe and life-threatening. Prompt diagnosis and treatment greatly reduces the chances that this might happen.

Unfortunately, DVTs can be missed, both by patients and their clinicians. The most common symptoms of a DVT include:

- Limb (arm or leg) pain and tenderness, often in the area of the calf
- Swelling of the limb (usually only one, but it can be in both in rare instances)
- Redness of the limb
- Increased temperature of the limb

As with many medical conditions, however, many patients who have a blood clot in an arm or leg don't present with all of the symptoms in a classic, reliable pattern. Therefore, sudden onset of pain or swelling and/or redness of an arm or leg should prompt a visit to the ER or doctor's office as quickly as possible. Also, certain conditions increase the likelihood of developing a blood clot:

- Prolonged periods of immobilization, like a long car or plane trip, or prolonged hospital stay
- Having a past history of a blood clot
- A strong family history of blood clots or certain blood clotting disorders
- Having cancer
- Taking birth control pills
- Smoking
- Recent injuries to the legs or certain types of surgeries (especially surgeries that result in prolonged immobilization afterwards)

So, if you develop leg pain or swelling, and any of the conditions mentioned above pertain to you, suspicion for a DVT should be even higher. Get to your doctor or the ER as quickly as possible.

Chapter 17

Neurologic

Change in Mental Status
Threat Level—Change in mental status: VERY HIGH-HIGHEST

A change in mental status refers to any of the following:

- A change in someone's ability to think clearly
- A change in someone's ability to process information
- Significant lapses in memory
- Disorientation (may not be able to identify self, time, or location)
- A change in personality
- A change in a person's level of alertness
- A change in a person's level of consciousness

A change in a person's mental status is always serious, but it is not always an emergency. There are an extraordinary number of possible causes of a change in mental status. Examples of medical conditions that can cause rapid, severe changes in mental status include:

- A very high or very low glucose level in a diabetic
- Overdose or poisoning
- Respiratory condition causing low oxygenation
- Infections

Examples of conditions that can cause slower changes in mental status include:

- Alzheimer's disease or other forms of dementia
- Depression or other forms of mental disease
- Metabolic conditions such as liver or thyroid disease

In general, how quickly someone requires medical attention for a change in mental status correlates well with the severity of the observed changes and how quickly the changes occur.

In other words, significant or severe changes in mental status that occur over a short amount of time—minutes to hours or days—are emergencies that require medical attention as quickly as possible, while minor or subtle changes that occur over weeks to months are rarely an emergency but should receive medical attention in the near future.

Seizures

Threat Level–Seizures: see below
Threat Level–Seizure that lasts longer than 5 minutes: HIGHEST

For someone who is not familiar or experienced with seizures, witnessing a seizure, especially a generalized or tonic-clonic seizure, as described below, can be a frightening experience.

A seizure may or may not represent a medical emergency. In this section, we will discuss what to do during a seizure and, of course, when to seek medical care.

First of all, there are many types of seizures. The type of seizure most people are familiar with is the generalized tonic-clonic seizure, where a person is not conscious or in control. During a tonic-clonic seizure, a person typically first stiffens and loses consciousness, followed by a period of jerking movements. There are *two important tasks* during a seizure:

- Protect the patient
- Time the seizure

To protect a person who is having a seizure:

- Move away any hard or sharp objects that could cause injury.
- Move the person away from any obvious area of danger, such as a ledge or staircase, if possible.
- If possible, lay the person on their side to prevent choking or aspiration.
- Place a pillow or other soft surface underneath their head.
- Do not place anything, including your hand, in the person's mouth.

A typical seizure may last from 1 to 3 minutes. It is important to time a seizure because a seizure that lasts longer than 5 minutes may signal an emergency situation, a prolonged seizure, which is known as status epilepticus. *Call 911 if a seizure lasts longer than 5 minutes.*

After a person has a seizure, they may be confused or groggy. They should be monitored until they are alert. Once a seizure has ended, then the decision must be made whether and when to seek medical attention.

The first question to ask following a seizure is whether the patient has a known seizure disorder or epilepsy. If a person has a known history of seizures or epilepsy and they appear to be recovering normally after a seizure, then the seizure is not an emergency and may not require further medical consultation.

If someone has a known history of seizures and is experiencing an increase in the frequency of their seizures or some other change in their typical seizure pattern, then they should seek medical care in the near future, usually within a few days to 2 weeks.

A first seizure, on the other hand, should be evaluated in an emergency room as soon as possible. The CDC lists the following reasons to consider a seizure an emergency and to call 911:

- The seizure lasts longer than five minutes without signs of slowing down, or if a person has trouble breathing afterwards, appears to be in pain, or recovery is unusual in some way.

- The person has another seizure soon after the first one.
- The person cannot be awakened after the seizure activity has stopped.
- The person became injured during the seizure.
- The person becomes aggressive.
- The seizure occurs in water.
- The person has a health condition like diabetes or heart disease or is pregnant.

Stroke
Threat Level–Stroke: HIGHEST

In the modern medical era, *stroke is the ultimate emergency* because appropriate treatment started within 3 hours may provide a fix, stopping and reversing the damage to the brain that is taking place.

The American Heart Association has developed a mnemonic for the warning signs of stroke: FAST.

Every person should know these warning signs of stroke (source: American Heart Association, Inc.):

- **F**ace drooping: Does one side of the face droop or is it numb? Ask the person to smile. Is the person's smile uneven?
- **A**rm weakness: Is one arm weak or numb? Ask the person to raise both arms. Does one arm drift downward?
- **S**peech difficulty: Is speech slurred? Is the person unable to speak or hard to understand? Ask the person to repeat a simple sentence, like "The sky is blue." Is the sentence repeated correctly?
- **T**ime to call 911: If someone shows any of these symptoms, even if the symptoms go away, call 911 and get the person to the hospital immediately. Check the time so you'll know when the first symptoms appeared.

Beyond FAST: Other Symptoms of Stroke You Should Know Include

(Again, courtesy of the American Heart Association):

- Sudden numbness or weakness of the leg, arm or face
- Sudden confusion or trouble understanding
- Sudden trouble seeing in one or both eyes
- Sudden trouble walking, dizziness, loss of balance or coordination
- Sudden severe headache with no known cause

If someone shows any of these symptoms, immediately call 911 or emergency medical services. The important point, once again, is that if a person shows any of the signs that they may be having a stroke, they must be evaluated (including a CAT scan of their head) and treated in an ER within 3 hours. That is not a lot of time.

It is not your job to diagnose the cause of a person's symptoms. It is your job to recognize the signs of a possible stroke and call 911 or go to the ER immediately.

And there it is, stroke in a nutshell.

A Remarkably Timed Stroke

Ann was a well-known poet. By the time I met her, she was in her eighties. We met when she became my patient, but we saw each other in public often as well. She was a delightful, intelligent woman.

Ann and I had both been asked to perform for one of our county library's periodic fundraisers. The entertainment at these fundraisers typically consisted of performances by local musicians. There was usually some type of theme to the event that shaped the performances. For this fundraiser, the theme was the Beatles.

I was going to perform the beautiful song "Across the Universe." I was outside warming up and fooling around with some of the other performers as Ann went on stage. She was one or two acts before me.

The event was held at beautiful Cacapon State Park, in a small lodge building near their lake and beach. Ann first read the lyrics to the well-known Beatles song "Blackbird." She followed with one of her own poems. The crowd applauded appreciatively as she finished her poem. With the audience still clapping, Ann fell to the floor. Something was wrong. Seconds later, the organizers of the fundraiser came to get me, telling me what had happened.

Just moments later, I was with Ann. She was on the floor but sitting up, and her eyes were open. I got down on the floor with her and asked what was wrong. She looked me in the eyes, and I thought she recognized and understood me.

Quickly, though, in a matter of just a few seconds, her eyes became unfocused. She couldn't answer me. Her face began to sag, and drool appeared at her lips. Her muscle tone weakened. We helped her lie back. Her left arm and leg became flaccid. It was obvious she was having a stroke. A major stroke.

Her breathing became irregular, and she exhaled in a gasp, spit coming out of her mouth. She stopped breathing. All of this had happened in what felt like about a minute. She was unresponsive. I checked for a pulse but could not find one.

I was in utter disbelief. Ann had been reading her own poetry just moments before, the crowd was applauding, and now she was dying in front of my eyes, while most of our community was sitting just a few feet away watching.

It had been years since I had been in a code blue situation, but my training kicked right in. Fortunately, a gentleman who identified himself as a military medic appeared at my side and began to assist. I asked someone to call 911 and told a friend to go to my car and get my black medical bag. Another friend was to call the main lodge at the park and try to find an AED (automated external defibrillator). I began chest compressions.

Periodically, we checked for a pulse but could still find none.

The AED arrived after about 10 minutes, and we applied the pads. There was electrical activity but still no pulse. In other words, Ann had pulseless electrical activity, which is not a shockable rhythm. The squad arrived, and Ann was taken out on a gurney. The crowd was in shock.

She was pronounced dead at our local hospital later that night.

She had died doing what she loved most, with the sounds of people's applause one of the last things that she would hear.

How's that for an exit?

What We Remember

The patient was an elderly woman who suffered from what appeared to be mild dementia. She lived alone. For months, I had been receiving reports from family, friends, and neighbors that she was doing terribly.

I had been seeing her regularly in the office, and when I raised these concerns with her, she always had the same response. "They think I'm crazy! But they're the ones who are crazy!"

At some point, however, she stopped coming in for regular appointments. I received a number of reports that she was very depressed and wouldn't leave the house. My nurse, Lindy, and I decided to have a look for ourselves and paid the patient a house call. She seemed her usual self. She was sassy!

We looked briefly around the home for signs that she was not taking care of herself. Her home was neat. Everything seemed in order. She appeared to be alert. She was clean, neatly dressed, and well fed. She was in good enough spirits.

I began to ask her some of the common questions we use to assess someone's mental status. She seemed to know that I was fishing for something, and her eyes narrowed.

"Who is the president?" I asked.

"George Washington" was her sarcastic reply.

"What is today's date?" I asked.

"Why do I care what the date is? I don't have anywhere to go!" she replied, again with a sarcastic tone.

I asked, "Can you name any of the schools you attended when you were younger?"

"Wouldn't you like to know!" she sassed.

She could not answer our questions, and she was trying to divert our attention with these answers. It was clear that her dementia was advancing. But we could also see that she seemed to be safe and well cared for.

We got up to leave. I said goodbye and walked out the door. My nurse remained a few moments longer, saying her goodbyes, and I heard the patient ask, "Who was that man?"

Lindy said, "That's the doctor, Dr. Hahn."

The patient hesitated for a moment and then asked, "Isn't he a Jew?"

That she remembered!

Lyme Disease?

This story involving a relatively subtle change in mental status stands out in my mind as one of the inspirations for writing this book.

The patient was well known to me, so I was in a good position to assess changes in his thinking or personality. He had begun to experience mental status changes many months before but had consulted a homeopath rather than coming to see me.

He had been told he had Lyme disease, an *E. coli* infection, and chronic fatigue and was receiving a number of remedies, none of which were effective.

I have evaluated and treated many people over the years for Lyme disease (including myself), so I am relatively familiar with the disease and its possible presentations. This seemed nothing like Lyme disease. There had been no characteristic rash or flulike illness at the outset. There was no significant joint pain. There were mental status changes that began and progressed slowly, primarily affecting language and writing ability. By the time the patient came to see me, he had lost the ability to write his name and even the alphabet.

The patient appeared outwardly fine to me, and we began with a pleasant and normal-seeming conversation. With a relatively simple test, the Mini Mental Status Exam, we identified some very impressive and concerning findings. When asked to write a sentence, the patient wrote out a symbol that looked like an M. I asked him to draw a clock face, and instead he drew a large number of squares ringing a circle. Despite outward normal appearances, it was obvious that something was very wrong.

We consulted a very good neurologist who identified what he called a classic case of Creutzfeldt-Jacob disease, a degenerative neurologic condition for which there is no known treatment or cure. The patient died from the condition within the year.

My point in telling about this case is to reiterate the point that your best bet when you suspect that something is seriously wrong is to consult a mainstream physician.

I believe that is your best chance for receiving an accurate diagnosis. Yes, physicians can be and are sometimes wrong in their assessments. And mainstream treatments sometimes fail or cause unintended consequences. But the odds that you will receive a correct diagnosis are best with a mainstream physician.

Once you receive that diagnosis and have discussed options for care, if you decide to go with a different type of care or to receive alternative care in conjunction with mainstream care, that is your decision, and you certainly have the right to make that decision. Your physician should respect your decision.

In this case, of course, even a correct diagnosis early in the course of the disease would have made no difference. Unfortunately, there is no effective treatment, mainstream or otherwise, for Creutzfeldt-Jacob disease.

Chapter 18

Skin

Dermatology, the branch of medicine concerned with conditions that affect the skin, is a rather broad topic. Diagnosis and treatment of most rashes would be, as they say, beyond the scope of this book.

In the section that follows we will focus on identification of skin conditions that require medical attention quickly because early treatment may be important.

As a general rule, it is important to note that any rash that is accompanied by the following symptoms or signs should receive prompt medical attention:

- High fever
- Significant pain or swelling of the area affected by the rash
- Difficulty breathing
- Feeling particularly ill or weak
- A rash that begins shortly after taking a medication, eating, or an insect sting (in the case of a sting, a concerning rash means a rash other than localized redness at the site of the bite)

Angioedema
Threat Level—Angioedema: VERY HIGH–HIGHEST

Angioedema (see Image 4) is a term used to describe rapid swelling of the skin, often of the face and/or hands, and also often of the mouth, tongue, and throat. It can be very dangerous because the swelling can be quite severe, and when it affects the mouth, tongue, or throat, it can block the airway.

Angioedema can be an allergic reaction. It can be a rare allergic reaction to a commonly used type of blood pressure medication called an angiotensin-converting enzyme (ACE) inhibitor. There is also a hereditary (nonallergic) form of angioedema.

Recognizing a case of angioedema (in other words, rapid swelling of any aspect of the mouth, tongue, or throat) is extremely important, so that treatment can prevent suffocation. Angioedema should be treated as an emergency. Immediate care can be lifesaving.

Cellulitis/Abscess
Threat Level—Cellulitis/Abscess: HIGH

Cellulitis (see Image 5) and abscesses (more commonly known as boils; see Image 6) are bacterial infections of the skin that require treatment as soon as possible. In the last decade there has been a rise in the number of skin infections related to the MRSA (methicillin-resistant *Staphylococcus aureus*) bacteria, which can often be more aggressive and more apt to spread, and therefore, appropriate treatment of these skin infections becomes even more important.

Cellulitis is characterized as spreading, often relatively large, areas of redness. The borders of a cellulitis infection are most often hazy, but can sometimes be quite sharp appearing. The skin affected by cellulitis is usually warm or hot, compared to normal skin temperature, and the rash is often stinging, itchy, or painful. The skin may swell. More worrisome is when a streak of redness extends up an arm or leg from an area of cellulitis, when a cellulitis infection begins to spread to the lymph system. Patients with cellulitis may feel ill. Patients who show signs of illness, such as a fever or flulike symptoms, require more aggressive treatment.

Cellulitis often begins when bacteria enter a cut or wound, even a very small one, but often, there is no obvious cause. Cellulitis sometimes develops in an area of trauma, such as a contusion, even when there is no obvious wound.

Cellulitis usually responds well to commonly used antibiotics. As MRSA has become so much more common in the recent past, it is important that doctors consider this as a possible cause and prescribe antibiotics that will work for these infections.

I would usually advise that any person with cellulitis receive treatment as soon as possible, preferably the same day that the infection becomes obvious. It is even more important that elderly or chronically ill people receive treatment as quickly as possible. Anyone who has cellulitis and is ill, or who has a skin infection that might affect a critical body part, such as the eye or nose, requires treatment most quickly.

An abscess, or boil, is an infection, usually of the skin (but an abscess can occur any place in the body), that becomes encapsulated, or walled off, filled with a thick cheesy or liquid pus.

An abscess may begin as an area of cellulitis but forms into a nodule or cyst that often has a white pustule (or pustules) with a tendency to burst and drain. They can be quite painful depending on their location and the amount and pressure of the pus that develops inside (I know, sounds disgusting, doesn't it?).

The treatment for an abscess is drainage. It may occur naturally but can be encouraged by applying warm compresses over the top, or a doctor can use a scalpel to incise and drain the abscess. What drains from an abscess is often smelly and disgusting (just the type of thing that delights doctor types).

Herpes
Threat Level–Herpes: HIGH

Most people are familiar with the appearance of cold sores (see Image 7), which are the result of an infection with a common form of the herpes virus. The same (or similar) virus is responsible for herpes outbreaks of the genitals. The rash of herpes often begins as itching or painful blisters (referred to as vesicles) over a red rash. On the mouth, there can be swelling, and the vesicles often transition into scabbing. People with a herpes outbreak often feel ill, though usually the illness is relatively mild and short-lived.

The reason it is important to be able to identify a herpes outbreak is that treatment with common antiviral medications, while not curative, if started within 2 to 3 days of the onset of the rash (the sooner the better), may shorten the course of the outbreak and decrease its severity.

Hives (Urticaria)

Threat Level–Hives: LOW
Threat Level–Hives associated with trouble breathing or wheezing, feeling sick to the stomach, dizziness, or weakness: HIGHEST

Hives (see Image 8) are usually a sign of an allergic reaction, but can be the result of infections, exposure to cold temperatures, or even stress. It is often difficult to identify the cause of hives.

Hives are often itchy and usually appear as one or more pink or red, smooth but slightly raised splotches (referred to as welts or wheals) on the skin. Hives are a type of rash that blanches (the skin color becomes temporarily lighter) when pressed or squeezed.

Hives are usually more annoying than dangerous. However, hives can be the first sign, or one of the signs, of a serious allergic reaction (see "Anaphylaxis"). Therefore, hives (especially around the face or mouth and usually appearing suddenly) that are associated with trouble breathing or wheezing, feeling sick to the stomach, dizziness, or weakness should prompt *immediate* medical attention.

Lyme Disease

Threat Level–Lyme disease: HIGH

I was fortunate to train in York, Pennsylvania, in the late 1990s, which was a time when Lyme disease was common in that region of the country. When I began practicing in western Maryland, we did not see any cases of Lyme disease for a few years. It became quite common after about 2002, and because I had seen a number of cases during my training, including my own case, I knew what I was seeing.

The tough part is that only 80 percent of cases of Lyme disease are accompanied by a rash.

When you do see the rash (see Image 9), however, which is in a large majority of cases, it should be unmistakable. Any large (average size 15 cm, which is about 6 inches) round or oval pink or red rash on a person who lives in an area where Lyme disease is prevalent should be considered a reason to go to the doctor. The characteristic rash is reason enough to treat with antibiotics. When the rash is present, testing for Lyme disease is not necessary, and can even be falsely negative.

In some cases, people have other symptoms, such as fever, headache, and joint pain, but in many other cases (such as my case), there were no symptoms besides the rash. In my experience, everyone has responded well to antibiotics.

I have seen no cases where someone who was treated early in the course of proven Lyme disease (they had the rash or a positive Lyme test) did not recover entirely. If you have the characteristic rash, it is usually not an emergency. You should receive antibiotics as soon as possible, but there is no emergency. The more symptoms you have besides the rash, the more quickly you should seek treatment.

Measles
Threat Level–Measles: HIGH

It's really a shame that I have to be writing about measles. Measles was a disease that was almost gone from America. Most doctors of my generation have never seen a case of measles. I have not.

Sorry, anti-vaxxers, but this one pisses me off. The measles vaccine, and all the typical infant vaccines (and most adolescent and adult vaccines, for that matter) are a modern miracle. I love them.

Alas, measles is back and we should all know what it looks like, primarily because it is incredibly contagious and easy to spread.

Unfortunately, measles begins as a cough and cold. Quickly, however, it becomes a really bad cold, with a severe cough, often associated with a high fever and redness (and drainage) affecting the eyes.

You may also note white spots inside the cheeks of a measles patient very early in the course of the disease. A good clinician will spot these and this can confirm the diagnosis of measles before the rash has started.

The rash of measles (see Image 10) only develops a few days into the illness, and the infection has already been spread. The rash consists of red spots and splotches that begin at the head and neck, and then spreads down the arms, the trunk, and eventually the legs. People with measles are infectious for about a week, beginning when they develop the first, nonspecific signs of illness.

Meningitis
Threat Level—Meningitis: VERY HIGH–HIGHEST

Bacterial meningitis is an infection that affects the lining of the brain, known as the meninges. There are various forms of meningitis. The most feared is a form of meningitis caused by a bacterium known as *Neisseria meningitidis*—hence the name meningococcal meningitis. This is still one of our most feared illnesses.

Symptoms of meningitis are well known by most people. A headache, fever, and feeling very ill are the most common early symptoms. Of course, those symptoms are common to many illnesses. Neck stiffness often accompanies meningitis. With meningitis, people appear quite ill.

The rash of meningococcal meningitis (see Image 11) is quite distinctive. At first, it appears like tiny bruises under the skin that can appear anywhere on the body. Later, the rash appears like dark bruises and splotches. What is most distinctive about the rash of meningococcal meningitis is that it will not fade (or blanch) if you press on it. Many rashes, when pressure is applied on top of them, will blanch, or turn pale or white. After pressure is removed, they will quickly fill in with color. The rash of meningococcal meningitis does not blanch.

This is an emergency. The more quickly the patient receives appropriate care, the more likely they are to live and to recover without permanent damage such as behavioral or intellectual disorders, or even deafness. Close contacts of the affected person may need treatment as well.

The most distinctive findings in someone who may have meningococcal meningitis is headache and fever, a very ill appearance (in my experience a person with meningitis is typically lying down and looks quite sick), neck pain or stiffness, and this nonblanching rash.

Get to an ER immediately if meningococcal meningitis is suspected.

Moles/Growths
Threat Level–Moles/Growths: LOW

When we are evaluating a mole or other type of skin growth, especially one that seems to be undergoing changes in size or appearance, we are really asking, "Is this mole cancerous, and if it is, is it melanoma?" There are three common forms of skin cancer:

- Melanoma
- Basal cell cancer (BCC)
- Squamous cell cancer

Of the common forms of skin cancer, melanoma (see Image 12) is the most worrisome. The other two are unlikely to spread to other parts of the body. Melanoma, especially if not caught early, can spread; it can be a very serious and deadly type of cancer under certain circumstances.

Fortunately, we have a relatively good guide to help us distinguish between noncancerous and cancerous types of moles and skin growths: the ABCDE system. Any mole that has any of the following ABCDE attributes should be evaluated by an experienced doctor as soon as possible:

- **A**symmetry: Noncancerous skin growths tend to be symmetric. That is, if you drew a line through the middle of the growth, the side on the left of the line would appear similar to the side on the right.

- **B**order: Noncancerous growths tend to have a smooth border, while a melanoma is more likely to have a jagged or irregular border.
- **C**olor: Noncancerous skin growths tend to be one color, whereas a melanoma is more likely to be a variety of colors.
- **D**iameter: Noncancerous skin growths tend to be smaller. Cancerous growths tend to be larger. Any skin growth over 6 mm in diameter (about the size of a pencil eraser) is more likely to be melanoma and should be evaluated.
- **E**volving: Noncancerous skin growths tend to remain the same size, shape, and color. Melanoma tends to grow and change size and shape relatively quickly.

Shingles
Threat Level–Shingles: HIGH

Shingles is an important rash to identify early because early treatment with antiviral medicines reduces the risks of developing a painful post-shingles syndrome.

Most people are familiar in some way with shingles. Shingles is the reawakening of the virus that causes chickenpox. After we are initially infected with chickenpox (or receive the chickenpox vaccine), the virus lies dormant in the nerves of the skin. At some point, typically in people over the age of 60 (shingles becomes more common the older we get), the virus reawakens in the form of the blistering rash that we know as shingles.

As most people also know, shingles can cause pain. The rash of shingles can be painful, but some people also continue to have pain well after the rash has healed. For a small number of these people, the pain can be quite severe and debilitating.

There are a number of key findings that help to distinguish shingles (see Image 13) from other rashes. First of all, the rash often begins as red splotches that soon develop blisters. Second, the rash of shingles can

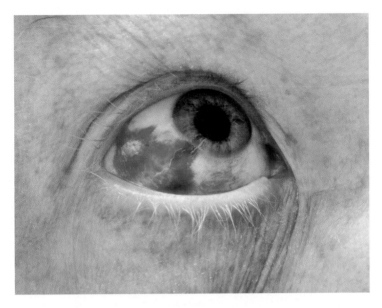

1. Subconjunctival hemorrhage (Credit: iStock.com/Steve Vanhorn)

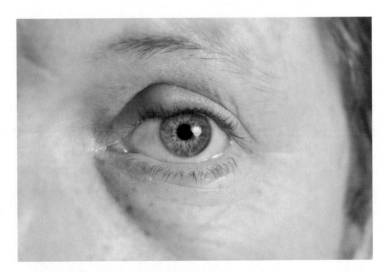

2. Sty (Credit: iStock.com/H_Barth)

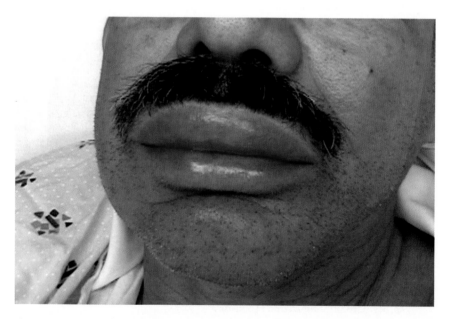

Right		Left
Gallstones Stomach Ulcer Pancreatitis	Stomach Ulcer Heartburn/ Indigestion Pancreatitis Gallstones	Ulcer Pancreatitis
Kidney stones Urine Infection Constipation	Pancreatiti Early Appendicitis Stomach Ulcer Inflammatory Bowel Umbilical hernia	Kidney Stones Diverticular Disease Constipation Inflammatory bowel disease
Appendicitis Constipation Pelvic Pain Groin Pain (Inguinal Hernia)	Urine infection Appendicitis Diverticular disease Inflammatory Bowel Pelvic pain	Diverticular Disease Pelvic pain Groin Pain (Inguinal Hernia)

3. Sections of the torso

4. Angioedema of lips (Credit: American Academy of Allergy, Asthma & Immunology)

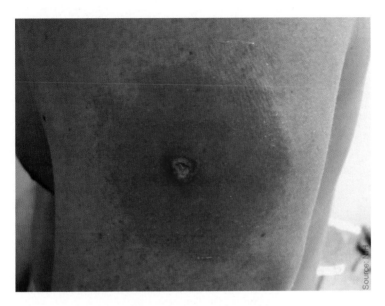

5. Cellulitis (Credit: National Institutes of Health)

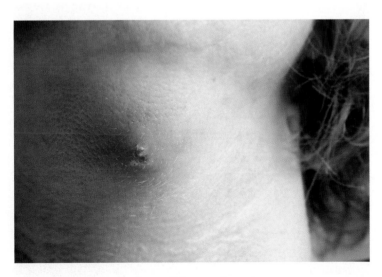

6. Abscess (Credit: iStock.com/MementoImage)

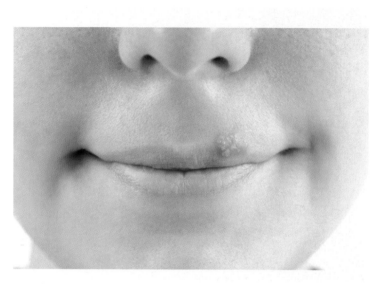

7. Cold sore (Credit: iStock.com/LeventKonuk)

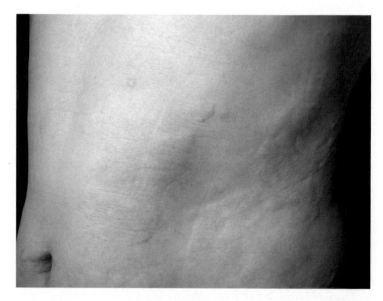

8. Hives (Credit: iStock.com/Mr_seng)

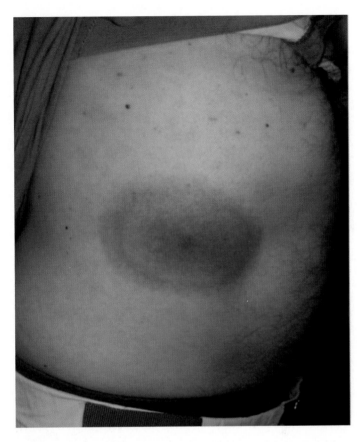

9. Lyme rash

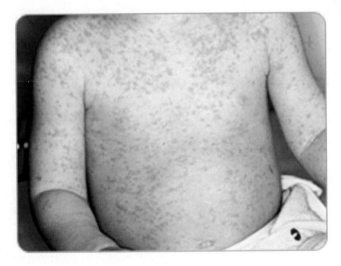

10. Measles (Credit: Waushara Argus)

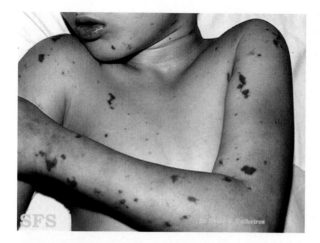

11. Meningococcal rash (Credit: Healthhype.com)

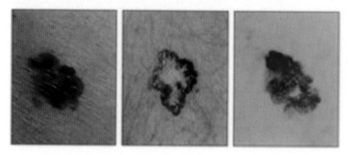

12. Melanoma (Credit: Healthwise Inc. & NCI Visuals)

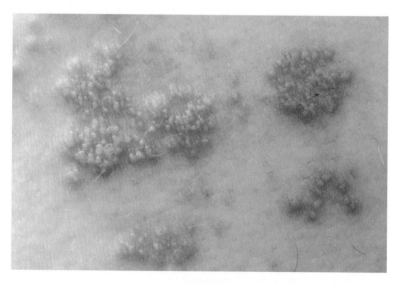

13. Shingles (Credit: iStock.com/clsgraphics)

OLD DAYS

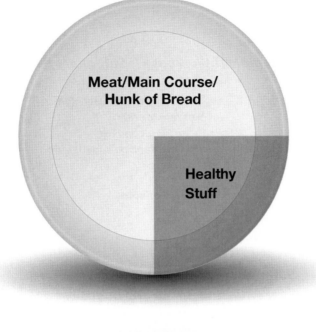

**Meat/Main Course/
Hunk of Bread**

**Healthy
Stuff**

TODAY

**Vegetables/Salad/
Fruit/Beans**
(Healthy Stuff)

**Healthy
Main Dish**

14. Plate illustration

Sample HIIT Workout #1: Stationary bike

1. Set the bike to a relatively high level of resistance.
2. Pedal for 60 seconds at maximum intensity. Repeat for a total of 5 sets.

Total workout time: 9 minutes

Sample HIIT Workout #2: Each exercise at maximal speed and intensity

1. Burpees for 45 seconds, rest for 15 seconds.
2. Jumping jacks for 45 seconds, rest for 15 seconds.
3. Favorite abdominal exercise for 45 seconds, rest for 15 seconds.
4. Run in place as quickly as possible for 45 seconds, rest for 15 seconds.
5. Burpees for 45 seconds, rest.

Total workout time: 4 minutes and 45 seconds

only be located on one side of the body. This is because the virus that causes shingles resides in the nerves of the skin, and these nerves begin in the spine and travel across the body, ending at the midline in the front of the body. Therefore, any rash that crosses over the middle of the body or affects both the right and left side of the body cannot be shingles.

The third thing that often can distinguish shingles from other rashes is pain. The shingles rash is often accompanied by stinging, burning, itching, and pain. Interestingly, those symptoms sometimes precede the rash! It is not uncommon for the pain to begin a few days prior to any sign of a rash.

Some people also feel ill with shingles, but that is less common.

So, a one-sided, blistering, painful rash is likely to be shingles.

If you think you might have shingles, get to the doctor as soon as you can. The earlier that medicine is started, especially if it is within 2 or 3 days from the first sign of the rash, the more likely it is to be effective. Medicine is not a cure for shingles, but it may shorten the course of the rash and decreases the likelihood of a post-shingles pain syndrome.

There are two special notes that you should also know about shingles. Shingles has a tendency to develop on the face, often on the forehead and around the eye. Shingles that affects the eye itself can be quite serious. It is especially important to identify shingles that might affect the eye early so that treatment can be started as quickly as possible.

Second, the shingles rash is contagious for those who are not immune to chickenpox. Anyone who might be susceptible to chickenpox, such as very young children who have not yet received the chickenpox vaccine, adults who never had chickenpox or received the vaccine, and those with impaired immune systems should not touch the shingles rash, as it can transmit chickenpox.

Finally, remember that prevention is key. There is a vaccine that can prevent most cases of shingles. It is recommended for people 60 years of age and older. As with many things in this country, though, it is expensive, running about $200. I always recommend that my patients check with their insurance prior to getting the vaccine. Because of the expense, many people do not end up getting this vaccine, unfortunately.

Stevens-Johnson Syndrome
Threat Level—Stevens-Johnson syndrome: VERY HIGH

Stevens-Johnson syndrome is a diagnosis that strikes fear into the hearts of all doctors because it is usually caused by a medication we prescribed, most often an antibiotic.

Stevens-Johnson syndrome is one form of a group of skin and mucous membrane reactions most often associated with recently started medications, but also with certain types of infections, known as toxic epidermal necrolysis (TENS). Severe cases may cause death.

People often begin to feel ill with common symptoms like fever and sore throat. Painful ulcers and blisters begin to form, most often affecting the mouth and lips, but sometimes also eyes, nose, genitals, and anus. A rash often affects the skin and can progress to blistering and peeling, almost like a severe burn or sunburn.

There is no specific cure for Stevens-Johnson syndrome, but in my experience, if the cause, usually a medication, most often an antibiotic, is stopped quickly, the symptoms are usually relatively mild and last only a short time.

The message is that if you are on an antibiotic or have started some other new medication and begin to develop pain and sores that affect the mouth, do not take the medication any longer and contact your physician immediately.

Serious cases are a dermatologic emergency and are often treated in burn units.

Toxic Shock Syndrome (TSS)
Threat Level—Toxic shock syndrome: HIGHEST

Thankfully, toxic shock syndrome is relatively rare (because it is a dangerous illness). Most people who are familiar with TSS remember back to the 1980s and 1990s when there were a large number of cases affecting young women who were using a super-absorbent tampon. When it was discovered that these tampons were the cause, they were removed from the market. Cases of TSS have become relatively rare since then.

TSS is a syndrome caused by two types of bacteria (*Staphylococcus aureus* and *Streptococcus pyogenes*) and usually results in a syndrome that includes a high fever, falling blood pressure, usually severe illness, and a red rash that can affect a very large area of the body and is often described as looking similar to a sunburn.

The reason that it is important to be able to identify TSS is that prompt treatment and especially removal of the source of the infection (such as a tampon) can be lifesaving.

My Mom and Melanoma

My mom was a healthy 78-year-old woman. I couldn't ever remember her being particularly ill. She had remained a teacher well into her seventies and had just retired. She had slowed down a little bit physically but was still as sharp as ever. She was the center of our good-sized family, as many moms are. My four siblings and I had done a rather poor job of providing her with grandchildren (there were only three), but her grandchildren were an incredible source of joy. I had never seen her as happy as when she was with them. It was sort of insulting, but I understood.

I have a picture of my mom on my desk in one of my exam rooms, holding my then two-year-old daughter. The smile on her face is the biggest smile I have ever seen.

As I remember it, her problems began early in the summer of 2001. My dad had found her passed out in the dining room. She recovered and saw her doctor soon thereafter. I had been in practice for about a year at that time. No one thought to contact me about this. I don't think that it would have made any difference anyway.

Then, on a Sunday in October, she suddenly lost partial vision in one eye. This they called me about. I was taking a nap during the afternoon, and my wife woke me and handed me the phone. It was my mom and dad.

"We think your mom has had a slight stroke," my dad said. I advised them to go to the ER, which they did. Appropriately, an MRI of her head was performed. Unfortunately, it was not a stroke. She had a number of large tumors in her brain. The radiologist thought that the appearance looked most like a brain metastasis from melanoma. In other words, she had melanoma that had spread to her brain.

She received whole brain radiation as a palliative treatment so that the brain tumors would not cause undue pain and suffering. There was little else to be done. About a month after receiving the radiation treatments, they began to affect her mental function. She was soon suffering from rather severe dementia as a result.

Not too long after that she had to be moved to a nursing home. In the nursing home, she fell and broke her hip. She would never walk again.

She died in late September 2002 in a hospice facility.

Mom's illness and eventual death provided any number of profound lessons for me both as a person and a physician.

First of all, if Mom could die, then so would I. I was thirty-nine years old at the time, the same age my mom was when I was born. I could clearly remember her when she was not much older than I was now. It didn't seem that long ago.

It became clear to me that the only defense against my mortality is to accomplish whatever I am meant to do. If we wait, it may be too late. Sad death, final moments filled with regret, is our greatest fear.

My passion at the time was getting patients to take better care of themselves. All day long, I was treating preventable conditions, such as diabetes and heart disease. The problem as I saw it was that physicians did not do enough to prevent these largely preventable conditions. I soon began a community effort called the Health Olympics, which was an attempt to get people to take better care of themselves.

As far as my mom's medical care had been concerned, I was hugely disappointed. I knew that there was not much that could be done to save her. She had a largely untreatable cancer. My disappointment was that there was no medical professional who took the responsibility to guide her care.

My dad had switched mom away from our long-time family doctor, upset that he had not made mom's diagnosis a few months earlier when she had passed out. This would not have made any difference. Once she had tumors in her brain, it was just too late. None of the other doctors that they saw, neither the specialists nor her primary care doctors, seemed to be willing or able to guide her care in an appropriate or even caring manner.

I swore that my practice would be different. We made it a point after that (in fact, it became a written goal) to care for our patients in the manner that we would hope our own family members would be cared for if they were ill. I believe, for the most part, that they are.

We have my mom to thank for that.

Chapter 19

Organizing Your Medical Information

In this brief section, you will learn to organize your medical history and describe your most important symptoms like a doctor! Knowing how to do this will enable you to communicate far better with your medical team—which could save your life!

I will also say this time and again: *be brief.* Save your *magnum opus* medical memoir for your English Lit class, or Facebook, or your diary. It's simple. The less you write, the more likely it is that it will be read. Everyone is busy. Doctors are even busier. Strive for quality over quantity.

Your Medical History

An organized medical history is the cornerstone of any medical relationship, and for good reason. A brief, well-organized medical history tells a medical professional everything they need to know about you as a patient. No, it doesn't impart to them what an incredible human being you are, but it creates a story of you as a patient that your medical team will understand, gives them key information they need to make important clinical decisions, and, most importantly, will help prevent their making mistakes when they treat you.

Your medical history may be the most important information that you share with your medical team. Fortunately, one of the first things they teach students in medical school is how to get a structured medical history from a patient.

And, believe it or not, all doctors are taught almost exactly the same structured medical history format. So, if you describe your medical history in New Jersey but then later end up in Oregon (or even Texas, believe it or not), everyone in the medical world you meet will be familiar with—and should be using—that same format! Well then, wouldn't it make sense for us to teach patients that same format? Then we could all speak the same language!

Here it is, the structured medical history:

- Past medical history (or diagnoses)
- Current medications and supplements
- Medication allergies
- Immunization history
- Social history
- Family history
- Hospitalizations and surgeries
- Health maintenance
- Other relevant information (this is not usually listed, but I added it!)

Carrying around, at all times, in whatever format (paper, electronic, etc.) suits you, a *brief* structured medical history, organized in this fashion, can save your life. Being ready to share this information at the beginning of any medical relationship—meeting a new doctor, going to the ER, having surgery, and so on—and further, keeping the information up to date by incorporating new information and any other changes, is one of the most important things you can do to optimize your health care. And, again, it could even save your life!

With that being the case, let's look at each category of the structured medical history, to describe each in more detail. Remember, though, brevity is the soul of wit—and a good medical history!

If your medical history goes over a page, you've either been unlucky or you're trying too hard. Keep it brief and to the point!

Past Medical History (or Diagnoses). Your past medical history is your history of important diagnoses. Another way to view the past medical history is all the significant things doctors have treated you for in the past. So here you would list all previous diagnoses like asthma, high blood pressure, diabetes, and specific cancers, for instance.

You don't need to list every minor diagnosis. For instance, it's not important to list that you had a minor cold virus last February. However, if you tend to suffer from one type of minor illness frequently, that is important. For instance, many women tend to have frequent urinary tract infections.

For each listed diagnosis, you may want to provide details (but keep it brief, please), such as:

- Year it was first diagnosed.
- Names of any other treating health-care practitioners (if there are any).
- Any other pertinent related information about you and your diagnosis. For instance, if you have high cholesterol but can't take statin cholesterol medications, that should be listed.

Women can also include their gynecologic history. In medicine, women are special! Men should not include a gynecologic history. A gynecologic history includes:

- Number of total pregnancies, births, living children, miscarriages, and surgical abortions
- Any other pertinent or interesting history regarding an individual pregnancy
- Age of first menstrual period
- Duration and frequency of periods
- Problems experienced related to menstrual periods
- Age when menstrual periods stopped

Current Medications and Supplements. A current, accurate medication list is critical. For all prescription medications and any common over-the-counter medicines include:

- Name of the medicine
- Dose or strength of the pill (i.e., "400 mg")
- How you take the medicine (i.e., by mouth, injection, nasal spray, etc.)
- How often you take the medicine (i.e., once per day, twice per day)

Medication Allergies. *These may be the most critical!* Your medication allergy list should include the name of the medicine and the reaction that you had to the medicine (i.e., penicillin, rash).

You may also want to list other specific allergies or adverse reactions you have to nonmedicine substances. For instance, if you have a reaction to latex, that should be listed here.

Immunizations. For anyone under the age of 18, a list of all immunizations, by date, is a good idea. For anyone older than 18, make sure to list, by date:

- Most recent tetanus shot
- Most recent flu shot
- Pneumonia shot history
- Shingles vaccine history
- Hepatitis B vaccine history
- HPV (human papillomavirus) vaccine history
- History of any other vaccines

Social History. This is where you may get to tell us what an amazing (or risk-taking) person you are. At its most basic, the social history should include:

- Current alcohol use: Just the most basic information, like how many drinks per day or week. Or maybe you're that rare patient that doesn't drink at all! If you have a history of significant alcohol abuse, or addiction, you should also list that in the past medical history section.
- History of tobacco use: Both smoking and smokeless tobacco, please.
- History of significant street drug use: Not important to tell us about what you did at Woodstock. But, rather, if you currently use any street drug, that is important to list. Hey, you folks in states where marijuana is legal, congratulations. But be safe, please!
- Caffeine use: Include coffee (my favorite form of caffeine), tea, soda, etc. By the way, I believe that coffee makes me smarter and better looking!
- Other: You may also want to list such things as your:
  - Current job or vocation.
  - Marital status.
  - Sexual history: Only the basics, such as gender preferences and number of partners (if you are comfortable relating that information).
  - Highest level of education.
  - General description of your eating habits (i.e., generally healthy, unhealthy, vegetarian, etc.).
  - General description of your exercise habits.
  - Pets: That's right! Animals may increase the likelihood of certain illnesses.
  - Hobbies: Here's where you can really shine!

Family History. We tend to view family history in three ways:

1. Pertinent medical conditions of "first degree relatives"—parents and siblings, especially for things like cancer, heart disease, diabetes, and mental disorders (because these tend to run in families).

2. Other medical conditions that tend to run in your family. For example, all the men on Dad's side have an extra nipple. Include especially interesting genetic conditions (because they are genetic!).

3. *Positive* family history (someone in your family had it) or *negative* family history (no one in your family had it) of certain key conditions. A positive or negative family history of these conditions may affect how we treat *you*!

   a. Colon cancer

   b. Prostate cancer (men only!)

   c. Breast cancer (mostly women!)

   d. Ovarian cancer (women only!)

   e. Heart disease and stroke

   f. Diabetes

   g. Depression

   h. Osteoporosis

Hospitalizations and Surgeries. Include the dates and the reason for the hospitalization or the name of the surgical procedure.

Health Maintenance. Include dates of latest cancer screenings:

- Colonoscopy or other colon cancer screening, such as stool blood testing
- Mammogram (women only)
- Pap smear (women only)

Other Information. You may want to include who can view your medical information and emergency contacts.

The History of the Present Illness: How to Tell Your Health-Care Team about Your Current Complaint

So you are concerned about a symptom you are having. You make an appointment with your doctor. What information should you tell them about your symptom(s)? In fact, what you tell your doctor, and how you describe your symptoms, may help (or hinder) a correct and timely diagnosis. In this brief section, we will teach you an effective method to describe your medical complaints.

In addition to being taught a format for a patient's past medical history, doctors are also taught a format for performing a medical interview that targets your current complaint or complaints. Having information in this standard format helps the physician in recognizing patterns that can indicate the nature of the patient's illness. We refer to that interview format as the *history of the present illness,* abbreviated as HPI.

What if patients actually knew this format, too? Wouldn't it help you to know what information regarding your problem(s) doctors want to know? Couldn't that help doctors and patients communicate better? What if you even came to the doctor's office or the hospital with the HPI all typed up and ready for review?

This format is extremely useful and easy to learn. You will note when you consider the details of the HPI format that it was really developed to describe pain, or an injury, but it can easily be adapted to almost any symptom.

The best way I can describe the HPI is that it is a narrative description of your symptom(s) or illness, or in other words, the story of your symptom(s). The HPI is best when it is as brief as possible and when it flows from start to finish like a story would. It should contain as much detail, or as I like to say, the flavor of what has been happening, as it takes to convey the story well.

It is often helpful to include in your story why you are concerned about your symptom(s), or what you are most concerned about. In other words, why is this symptom important to you? Is there a reason that you sought medical care other than just wanting to know the medical significance of the issue? For instance, if you are having headaches and your mom and grandfather both died of an aneurysm, this may be really important context to share with your physician. Brevity is still a virtue, however.

The HPI should contain, at a minimum, the following content (if applicable):

- Chief complaint
- Duration
- Severity
- Location (for a complaint of pain, or an injury or rash)
- Context
- Quality
- What makes it better or worse
- Associated signs and symptoms
- Treatments

Chief Complaint. The chief complaint is a very brief statement of why you have come to the doctor. It should be as few words as possible (i.e., "cough," or "right shoulder pain").

Duration. The duration, or onset, of a symptom is pretty basic, but also very helpful. When did the problem begin, roughly? You may also note if the symptom(s) began suddenly or progressed gradually.

Severity. This is most relevant for a pain-related complaint. How bad, or how intense, is the pain? For pain, the 0–10 rating scale is useful, with 0 being no pain, and 10 being pain so bad you wish we would just amputate! We recognize that these things are subjective. You may also want to note if the pain or intensity varies in some way.

Location. This also really only relates to pain or to an injury. So you may have a sprained right ankle. However, "Location" isn't terribly appropriate to include if your complaint is a cough!

Context. The context of a symptom describes where and when it tends to occur. What are the circumstances that tend to trigger the symptom(s)? So the context of a sprained ankle could be, "I was table-dancing drunk at Julio's, and I fell off the table, injuring my ankle."

Quality. This is another category that primarily relates to pain. The quality, or character, of pain can be sharp or dull. It can be burning or electric, and so forth. Be creative, but also try to be accurate, and, of course, *brief*!

Timing. Is there a pattern or timing to when your problem tends to bother you? It can be constant (but is it really?), or only during the day, only at night, or it can come and go. Sometimes, there may be no pattern at all!

What Makes It Better or Worse. We in the medical fields call this the "modifying factors," which means what tends to make the problem better or worse. For instance, rest, being off work or school, tends to make all my patients better, whereas work or going to school tends to make them worse. Can you believe that?

Treatments. What crazy treatments have you tried and what happened when you tried them? Be honest! If you took your wife's antibiotics (or pain pills), 'fess up!

Associated Signs and Symptoms. This is kind of a catch-all category. Just try to think in the area of the problem, what else is going on? For instance, if you sprained your ankle table dancing, is there swelling or redness of the ankle?

I would also like to advise that if you have what you think may be a significant or complicated issue, make every attempt to schedule an appointment to focus on that issue alone. Many patients who have regularly scheduled appointments for chronic issues, such as high blood pressure or diabetes, like to save their other complaints for their next regularly scheduled appointment. While most doctors are used to and quite capable of handling multiple complaints, this makes it challenging to give the additional, and often more concerning, complaint the attention it deserves.

Similarly, if you are concerned about a significant issue (or issues), it is not the best idea to schedule a "physical" to discuss them. A "physical" usually implies what medical professionals refer to as a "well visit" and has certain clinical (and insurance billing) implications and responsibilities. Once again, an appointment like this may make it more challenging to give the most important issues the attention they require.

Example of a Structured Medical History

Past Medical History
- Hereditary spherocytosis, 1965
- High blood pressure, 2002
- High cholesterol, 2005
- Sarcoidosis, 2008; see pulmonologist Dr. Perry
- Seasonal allergies, 1990

Current Medications and Supplements
- Amlodipine 5 mg by mouth in the morning
- Atorvastatin 20 mg by mouth at night
- Advair 250/50 one inhalation two times per day
- Albuterol 2 puffs every 4 to 6 hours as needed
- Flonase nasal spray 2 sprays per nostril every day

Medication Allergies
- Penicillin: trouble breathing, rash

Immunization History
- Tetanus shot 2010
- Flu shot October 2015
- Hepatitis B vaccine series 2009

Social History
- Alcohol: 1 beer per day

- Tobacco: none
- Recreational drugs: none that I'll tell you about
- Caffeine use: coffee, of course, 2 cups in the morning
- Job: supermodel
- Marital status: married to first wife
- Eating: I can't eat gluten
- Exercise: I run 20 miles per day
- Pets: 2 dogs that we treat like children
- Hobbies: stamp collecting

Family History
- Colon cancer: no family history
- Prostate cancer: father, age 60
- Breast cancer: no family history
- Ovarian cancer: no family history
- Heart disease and stroke: mother, heart attack, age 80
- Diabetes: no family history
- Depression: no family history
- Osteoporosis: no family history

History of Hospitalizations and Surgeries
- Pyloric stenosis repair, 1963
- Right wrist fracture repair, 1993
- Partial thyroid removal, 2007

Health Maintenance
- Colonoscopy, 2013: normal

Other Relevant Information
- Emergency contact: Robert Redford 240-878-9767

Example of HPI

My chief complaint is a rash, joint pain, and fevers.

My symptoms began about a week ago when I started to feel tired and my joints began to ache. The next day I began to feel like I had a fever and started having a headache. I have continued having those symptoms off and on every day since. My knees began to ache a couple of days ago as well. Yesterday I noticed a large round rash on my right thigh.

I am concerned because my sister had a terrible case of Lyme disease, and when I told her about my symptoms, she said I sounded just like she did. I have been out hunting lately, and I get ticks all over me, and I know that Lyme disease is pretty common around here.

The severity of my symptoms varies, but the headache has been intense at times. The headache usually starts in my forehead, but when it gets bad, it affects my whole head. The pain of the headache is dull. Nothing that I know of makes my symptoms worse. I feel better when I rest and for a little while after I take ibuprofen. I have been using the ibuprofen two or three times per day.

The only other things I can think of are that when the headache is at its worst, my stomach gets upset also.

PART 2

The Miracles of Twenty-First-Century Medicine

Taking Advantage of Modern Preventive Medical Care

"Isn't all medicine poison?" This was the question posed to me by a long-time patient. The question exemplifies an extremely common attitude held by many people today—that modern medicine is bad for you.

If you are someone who believes that prescription medicines are poison, or that modern medicine is bad for you, then it is very important that you read this section of *Staying Alive*. Here I argue that quite the opposite is true. More specifically, that two types of treatments—childhood immunizations and many of the medications prescribed for our most serious and common chronic diseases (high blood pressure, high cholesterol, heart disease, and type 2 diabetes)—are incredibly safe and highly effective. These treatments, along with healthy eating and regular exercise, are the best ways we know to protect your health.

In fact, they constitute what should be viewed as a true miracle of modern science and medicine.

My purpose in writing about this is not just to highlight the benefits of these therapies. That has been done, and the information is widely available (though it continues to be debated). More importantly, I would like to try and shift the focus of the conversation.

The starting point of the conversation needs to be this—*that the biggest threats to our health today are infectious diseases and the big three killers:*

heart disease, diabetes, and cancer. Having safe and effective treatments for these conditions, therefore, is of the utmost importance.

In 1900, the number one killer in the United States was infectious disease. Because of improvements in sanitation, the development of antibiotics, and the effects of immunizations, that is no longer the case. Today, heart disease, stroke, cancer, and diabetes are the number one causes of death (I am purposefully skipping over accidents and suicides, by the way). Together, they account for 43 percent of all deaths.

The next point that must be emphasized is that, despite the beliefs held by some to the contrary, *these therapies are incredibly safe.* The safety of childhood immunizations and the medications used to treat high blood pressure, high cholesterol, heart disease, and diabetes have been thoroughly and rigorously researched, and that research is ongoing. They have extraordinarily well-documented safety profiles.

What is most unfortunate is that the fear generated by the controversies surrounding these therapies keeps many people from taking advantage of one of the best lines of defense we have in fighting the most common and serious diseases that are likely to sicken, and even kill, many of us.

Put as simply as possible, eating healthy and exercising regularly, along with keeping children up to date with recommended childhood immunizations, and being monitored for and, if necessary, treated for high blood pressure, high cholesterol, heart disease, and diabetes, is the best way we know today to improve our health-related odds.

The attitude expressed by my patient's comment, that medication is poison, is rooted in certain valid and important concerns. That is what makes this a complicated topic. Because of the impact that infectious diseases once had on the lives of so many children, and the extreme impact that high blood pressure, high cholesterol, heart disease, and diabetes currently have on the lives of so many adults, this is a topic that is well worth discussing, in an effort to clarify those concerns and place them in a proper perspective.

It should be noted that I have no financial ties to the pharmaceutical industry. I receive no money for prescribing any medication. I accept no gifts from the pharmaceutical industry. As a result, I am not popular among the group of pharmaceutical reps that visit my practice.

Also, all treatments have limits, and all treatments have potential adverse effects. No vaccine or medication is 100 percent effective, and none is entirely free of potential adverse effects.

In addition, medical errors can be (and all too often are) made in administering even the best treatments. Used inappropriately, any treatment can result in harm. However, used appropriately and with proper caution, immunizations and the medications we will be discussing here are safe and remarkably effective.

Immunizations

I am not sure it is possible to reason with many anti-vaccinators. I view it as part of my job and part of my responsibility to try, however.

For the sake of brevity, I will limit the conversation to childhood vaccinations. It is not that I do not favor adult vaccination (I am a fan of adult vaccines as well). Including adult vaccines, however, makes this a much more complicated discussion that is best saved for another place and time.

Let me begin by offering a number of olive branches of sorts.

First of all, it is only with great humility that I make any medical recommendation. The reality and complexity of science and medical care is such that ideas we hold true one day may be disproven the next. One must always believe that it is possible, even if it is highly unlikely, that the benefits of vaccines are overstated and the risks understated. The huge weight of a huge body of evidence and experience, however, argues that immunizations are effective and safe.

Similarly, I understand, respect, and share grave concerns about the possibility that pharmaceutical companies, who have billions of dollars of profits on the line, overstate both the benefits and safety of their products, and may even hide or misrepresent key data regarding such issues. It has happened.

The immunizations that we administer in my office represent a cost, not financial gain. Though patients might not be aware of this, physicians' offices must purchase immunizations. In my practice, this represents a huge expense (it is the number two expense behind salaries). The reimbursement a physician receives from insurance companies for administering an immunization barely covers, and is often less, than the cost. In other words, I do not make money from immunizations. So from that perspective, you can trust my recommendations.

I believe that immunizations are *the single most important development in science and medicine in the history of the world to date and a true miracle of our times.* Vaccines prevent almost six million deaths annually worldwide.

The science supporting the effectiveness and safety of vaccines is convincing. The major safety risks referenced by most anti-vaccinators have been debunked time and again. Are they 100 percent safe? Almost!

In a very thorough 2011 review of the potential adverse effects of vaccines performed by the highly respected Institute of Medicine, vaccines were once again confirmed to be safe, and serious adverse reactions were found to be extraordinarily rare.

My experience as a physician supports this evidence. I have been a practicing physician for eighteen years, and I have never had a patient diagnosed with or die from polio, measles, German measles, tetanus, or diphtheria. Nor has a patient ever had a serious reaction to any immunization, and my staff has administered many thousands over the years (I acknowledge that serious reactions do occur, but they are extraordinarily rare).

Vaccines enable me and all of the physicians of my generation who practice in America and see children to be great pediatricians owing to the fact that we never see most of the serious infectious diseases that were a mainstay of the previous era. These diseases once killed many, many children.

Today, we can be complacent about the topic of immunizations owing to their great success in reducing serious illness. That success extends even to those who do not vaccinate, owing to "herd immunity." Herd immunity refers to the fact that when most members of a community are immunized, even those who do not receive immunizations receive the benefits because fewer people become infectious (and are therefore able to transmit the disease).

I was fortunate to work for many years with a colleague, Dr. Donald Straus, a wonderful pediatrician and good friend, who began his career in 1950, before there were immunizations for most of the serious infectious diseases that commonly afflicted children. Don told me many stories about the anguish of taking care of young patients who died or were severely maimed by the infectious diseases of the day.

I spoke to Don's wife, Selma, recently, and she recounted a number of stories. "I remember one beautiful, beautiful baby under a year old, admitted to the hospital in Frederick, Maryland, with measles. She became a vegetable. Unfortunately, she lived! She had been such a beautiful baby. That family suffered for years and years. I guess they still are."

Selma continued, "During the summers, my parents took us to the Catskill Mountains to get us out of the city because of polio. I had a teacher in second grade that I loved. I used to visit her until I graduated high school. She had a son who had polio. He survived it, but he was wheelchair bound. He was seven or eight years old when that happened."

I have no such stories to tell. Most likely, neither do you. That is because immunizations are so profoundly successful. Once again, I will say it. This is a miracle.

I won't spend a lot of time arguing the facts. This is a well-worn path, and I don't think there is any point that I can make that has not already been made time and again.

The choice not to immunize is an emotional one. It is about whom and what you choose to believe in a complicated and conflicted world. Everyone is entitled to make their own decisions regarding their own health care. However, the choice not to immunize affects others as well.

I will mention one caveat when it comes to immunizations (which I believe applies to all medical treatments). I advise caution with immunizations when they are new. In general, I am very cautious with any new immunization when it is first released.

Additionally, while I am a great fan and advocate for immunizations, I believe that some of the mandatory aspects of our immunization policies have been too heavy-handed. For instance, when the vaccine for human papillomavirus (HPV) was released in 2006, it was immediately mandatory in some states. Even though I am an advocate for the HPV vaccine, I felt that making this particular vaccine mandatory when it was brand new was inappropriate for a number of reasons. It certainly felt that this approach was motivated, at least in part, by a push for profits over safety and common sense. It tarnished the reputation of the HPV vaccine, which still is not being given in great numbers (partly because of the cost, and partly due to the fact that HPV is a sexually acquired infection, I believe).

What is truly unfortunate is that the ongoing arguments over the safety of childhood immunizations divert attention from what should be the real focus today: how to improve childhood immunization rates. Typical of many practices, our small office struggles to afford and administer immunizations. The chief reason is that the number of childhood (and adult) vaccine regimens has greatly expanded and grown more complicated over the years. There are currently 13 total immunizations suggested for children between the ages of 0 and 18 years of age. The costs and time involved in purchasing, maintaining, and administering all of these is staggering and prohibitive for many doctors' offices.

Many years back, when there were but a few childhood vaccines, it made sense and was simple for doctors to purchase and administer them. A far better approach today would be to provide vaccines at no cost to medical practices and also make them far more accessible to everyone through public health clinics.

Also, I wish the complicated regimens recommended today could be simplified.

My recommendation is to get your children immunized. Immunizations are a true miracle of modern health care. Take advantage of the miracle and be thankful for it. Fear the diseases that used to kill and maim thousands of children in the United States every year—not their cure.

Preventive Medications for Chronic Conditions

The burden of suffering and the financial impact associated with our most common chronic diseases—heart disease, type 2 diabetes, high blood pressure, and high cholesterol—are immense. Heart disease is the number one killer in the United States today. According to the Centers for Disease Control and Prevention, almost 1 in 3 adults will develop high blood pressure and high cholesterol, two of the most important risk factors for developing heart disease. Between the years 1980 and 2014, the incidence of diabetes in adult Americans more than doubled. These conditions are largely preventable through exercise and healthy eating; they are also now highly treatable with medication.

And yet it is common for my patients to say that they "hate medicine." Many take this notion substantially further and will do anything to avoid taking a long-term prescription medication or just refuse outright. If they do agree, they are always looking for a reason to stop their medications. These same patients also tend to experience side effects from prescription medications in far greater numbers than one would normally expect.

The opposite should be the case. I would go so far as to say that many people who get treated with medication for high blood pressure and high cholesterol may, in fact, be better off than those who do not. In my practice, the majority of strokes that have taken place over the past ten years have occurred in patients who were never treated with blood pressure or cholesterol medications, either because their numbers were not consistently high enough or because they resisted treatment. The medications used to treat such common conditions as high blood pressure and high cholesterol, as well as many of the medications (but not necessarily all) used to treat heart disease and diabetes represent a true modern miracle for health and medicine.

Rather than dread the notion of using these medications, we should take heart that we live in an era where we have discovered how to care so well for the most common, and most commonly dangerous, chronic medical conditions.

I think there is value in examining the underlying reasons that people fear prescription medications to such an extent.

At the heart of this issue, I think, are our fears of growing old and our denial of death and dying. The Baby Boomer generation is the first to be raised with an expectation (rather than hope) that they should live a long, healthy life, largely free of disease. Aging, being ill, and dying do not fit comfortably with these expectations. It is not entirely unrealistic to believe in this notion. It is not yet the reality experienced by many people either, though.

A diagnosis such as high blood pressure or heart disease, and the subsequent recommendation to take medication, is subtly viewed by many as a sign of aging, and of our mortality. It is a label of sorts that places us among a group we don't want to be part of.

The irony is that treating these conditions is one of the best ways we know to delay the effects of aging and prevent premature death.

Many people simply do not trust the American medical establishment. People's hesitance to trust the recommendations and research results of pharmaceutical companies, who stand to make billions of dollars from even one blockbuster medication, is based on valid concerns. One should always take any recommendation made by a pharmaceutical company with a grain of salt, look to more objective research (performed by researchers who do not benefit directly and monetarily based on the results of their work), and wait until there are multiple studies showing similar results before accepting research claims. It is completely valid, necessary, and healthy to question the safety and effectiveness of any medication, especially one that is new. The medical community encourages this and actively participates in the process.

However, the great weight of a great deal of relatively independent research, supported now by years of clinical experience, shows the benefits and safety of using medications to treat the most serious common chronic medical conditions: high blood pressure, high cholesterol, heart disease, and diabetes.

As I tell my patients, I am not here just to put them on medicine. My job is to lower their risks of serious disease and premature death as much as possible. Used appropriately and cautiously, and monitored regularly for effectiveness and adverse effects, the medications used for these common chronic conditions are the best ways we know to do this.

In my practice, I take care of many, many patients with high blood pressure, high cholesterol, heart disease, obesity, and diabetes. Many of those patients do not maintain the best diet (despite my urgings). Nor do they exercise as they should. And yet, even in the very short span of time that I have been in practice, over the past fifteen to twenty years, I have seen the face of medicine and patient care change dramatically as a result of the medicines and protocols used to treat these extremely common, but potentially deadly, chronic diseases. In my practice, I no longer see heart attacks or strokes (and many other conditions that result from uncontrolled blood pressure, cholesterol, and diabetes) in any way near the numbers that I used to see (many of my physician colleagues tell me the same thing). This is not because my patients take better care of themselves than other doctors' patients (I wish it were). I believe it is because I was trained to care for these chronic conditions as a regular part of my practice, and because the treatments and protocols that have been available over the past fifteen to twenty years (and are continually being refined) have made such a profound difference.

Still, many legitimate, complicated scientific questions and controversies exist regarding the best use of medications and their ultimate clinical effects. It is important that we continually refine our knowledge.

What is truly fascinating is that many people will ingest incredible quantities of what they consider "natural" remedies and supplements without questioning their effects or safety to any significant extent. "Natural" remedies receive little to no scrutiny and are assumed to be safe by virtue of their being "natural."

A natural remedy, loosely speaking, is one that is of natural origin. Of course, many prescription medications fit the loose description of being "natural," and many alternative and complementary remedies are clearly not "natural."

Nor are all natural substances safe. Mushrooms are natural and can be poisonous. In fact, the natural world is filled with dangerous and lethal substances.

On the other hand, many prescription medications are derived from nature. Digoxin, aspirin, female hormones, insulin, and penicillin (lots of antibiotics, in fact) were initially derived from natural substances. Angiotensin-converting enzyme (ACE) inhibitors, a very commonly used and effective type of blood pressure medication, are synthetic copies of a type of snake venom.

It needs to be noted that companies that manufacture and sell "natural" remedies are also businesses, motivated by the potential for huge profits, and have the same incentives as the companies that produce prescription medications to exaggerate the benefits and safety of their products. "Natural" remedies should be subjected to the same scrutiny regarding their benefits and safety as prescription medications.

It is useful to look at each of the four chronic diseases—high blood pressure, high cholesterol, heart disease, and diabetes—and the medications used to treat them.

High Cholesterol and the Statin Cholesterol Medications

No class of medications provokes more fear or carries more negative lore than the statin cholesterol medications, so we might as well deal with them first. "My friend/neighbor/family member told me horror stories about those medicines" is a frequent comment in my office.

Medicines like atorvastatin (trade name Lipitor), simvastatin (Zocor), rosuvastatin (Crestor), and pravastatin (Pravachol) are extraordinarily commonly prescribed medications.

Here's what you need to know about the statins:

1. **They are incredibly safe.** In 2001, still the early years of statin use, cerivastatin (the first statin, brand name Baycol) was removed from the market after it was found to be associated

with serious muscle conditions. This touched off a wave of panic and fear about this class of medications that persists today.

Fear of muscle disease, in addition to fears about liver toxicity, increased risk of developing diabetes, and memory concerns have dogged the statins.

Here is the most important information that has come to light over the past few years about the statin cholesterol medications: they are very safe—much safer than we had previously thought.

The US Preventive Services Task Force, which I consider one of the most conservative organizations that makes recommendations regarding clinical practices, recently completed an extremely thorough evaluation of the statin cholesterol medications. "Statin therapy was not associated with increased risk of withdrawal due to adverse events, serious adverse events, any cancer, new-onset diabetes; myalgia, or elevated aminotransferases. Evidence on the association between statins and renal or cognitive harms was sparse, but did not clearly indicate increased risk. Few serious adverse events were reported."

In other words, statins are safe. Statins are now felt to be so safe that it is no longer recommended that doctors follow a patient's liver function tests when they are using statins, and statins are even recommended to lower the risks for people with certain liver conditions.

2. **Statins are effective in both preventing and treating cardiovascular disease.** In the same comprehensive review by the US Preventive Services Task Force quoted above, the report also stated, "In adults at increased cardiovascular risk but without prior cardiovascular events, statin therapy is associated with reduced risk of all-cause and cardiovascular mortality and cardiovascular events."

In other words, statins are both safe and effective.

3. **Who benefits from the statins?** This is the most important question regarding the statin medications. It is very well

established that statins represent an incredible advance in the treatment of patients *with known heart disease.*

The real question is, which people *who do not have known heart disease* can benefit from using the statins?

The answer is that the more cardiac risks you have, the more likely you are to benefit from a statin. If you are a thin runner and conscientious eater with no family history of heart disease and no stress in your life, then it is less likely that a statin will lower your risks much further. If, on the other hand, you are overweight, don't exercise, smoke, and have a family history of heart disease in a first-degree relative, it is very likely that a statin will lower your risks substantially.

The difficulty is in determining each person's individual risk. The traditional known risk factors for heart disease—such as high blood pressure, obesity, lack of physical activity, poor eating choices, and a family history of heart disease—are helpful, but not perfect, in determining a person's actual risk. It is hard to know reliably, for instance, how badly an individual person's eating affects their actual risks. Even more, it is impossible to estimate how much stress, another known but hard-to-quantify risk factor, affects an individual.

Until we determine a better way to estimate an individual's cardiac risk, the American College of Cardiology, in their 2014 update regarding use of statins, recommends four circumstances where a statin is of benefit: anyone with known heart disease; people aged 40 to 75 with known diabetes or calculated 10-year risk of heart disease of 7.5 percent or higher; people with low-density lipoprotein (LDL) cholesterol of 190 or higher.

4. **Statins can cause reversible muscle pain or muscle weakness.** Every person who uses a statin medication should be aware that it is not uncommon for them to cause muscle pain or muscle weakness. This may affect up to 25 percent of statin users at some point, though exact figures are difficult to come

by. These effects are reversible by stopping the medication. If you experience an uncommon amount of muscle soreness or weakness while you are taking a statin medication, contact your physician. It is usually possible to find a statin medication and dose that do not cause these symptoms.

In summary, you should not fear statin cholesterol medications. Fear heart disease, which is the disease most likely to kill you. Be thankful we have treatments that protect us from heart disease and hope that you are one of the people that statins can help.

High Blood Pressure

Besides healthy eating and regular exercise, successfully treating high blood pressure with medication is the most important, reliable, and well-studied way we can lower our risks of heart attack and stroke.

Comprehensive recommendations for the treatment of high blood pressure were recently updated in a much anticipated report known as the JNC 8 (Report of the 8th Joint National Committee), which has been the gold standard for recommendations regarding the treatment of high blood pressure.

In their report, the JNC 8 cited the results of many well-done large-scale studies on the effects of treating high blood pressure with medication. The research shows a consistent large (impressively large) reduction in the number of cases and the rate of death from stroke, heart disease, and heart failure.

Used properly and appropriately monitored, the medications most often used today for the treatment of high blood pressure are quite safe. The JNC 8 made specific recommendations regarding the best medication options.

From a patient's perspective, the most important issues are cost and side effects. It should usually be possible today to treat patients' blood pressure with less expensive, generic medicines. Try to steer clear of the newer brand name medicines, as they may cost substantially more than the generic versions but offer no greater clinical benefit.

Medicines used to treat high blood pressure can have bothersome side effects. The objective should be to find a medicine, or combination of medicines, that is well tolerated.

The current battle concerning blood pressure treatment concerns optimal blood pressure targets. Recent well-known and highly regarded guidelines suggest that for people over the age of 60, an upper limit of 150 may be an acceptable goal for systolic (the top number of a blood pressure reading is the systolic pressure, while the bottom number is referred to as the diastolic pressure) blood pressure (140 has been the accepted limit for many years). This recommendation has been disputed by many researchers and a number of subsequent studies. On the other hand, lowering the systolic blood pressure to much lower than 120 may cause more harm than benefit. These are legitimate questions regarding the treatment of high blood pressure, and they will continue to be debated.

Heart Disease

Heart disease is the number one killer in the world. Having effective treatment for heart disease, therefore, is of paramount importance.

The advancements made in the treatment of heart disease, be it medications, cardiac surgery, or cardiac catheterization and angioplasty, constitute a true, and very welcome, revolution in modern care.

I have always found cardiology to be the most impressive medical specialty because of its great success and continual improvements in the ability to care for people with such serious disease. I take care of many patients diagnosed with heart disease. But today, owing to the success of modern therapy, I have no patients whose conditions have deteriorated to active congestive heart failure, which previously dominated the care of these patients in my practice. Our ability to prevent heart attacks, treat them when they occur, and prevent the development of congestive heart failure is dramatically improved.

Four types of medication form the cornerstone of modern treatment of heart disease: beta blocker blood pressure medications, ACE inhibitor blood pressure medications, the statin cholesterol medicines, and aspirin and other types of blood thinners. These medications have proven themselves time and again as safe and very effective

Except for the newer blood thinners, it should be possible to treat patients with generic medications that are affordable. It should also be possible to find a combination of treatments that are well tolerated.

Type 2 Diabetes

In just a little over two decades, type 2 diabetes has gone from a disease that often resulted in blindness, heart disease, kidney failure, and amputations to a much more manageable condition. Properly treated patients have far fewer of these dreaded complications.

I take care of hundreds of patients with type 2 diabetes. It is a major focus of my practice (as are all of the chronic diseases we are discussing here). In stark contrast to what I witnessed during my training in the 1990s, and my earlier years of practice, despite treating a great many more patients with type 2 diabetes, I have no diabetic patients currently who are blind, none in dialysis, and none who have lost a limb as a result of their disease. To a large extent, most of these patients live free of significant complications from their disease. This constitutes a modern miracle!

Here is the conundrum in using medications to treat type 2 diabetes. We know that controlling a diabetic's blood sugar results in incredible reductions in the complications associated with diabetes. But of the myriad medications now available, only one, metformin, has been shown to lower the rate of death and complications in patients with type 2 diabetes.

The irony here is that it may not be the treatment of high blood sugar that creates much of the improvements we see in patient outcomes associated with type 2 diabetes. Controlling blood sugar levels is only one aspect of the treatment, though. Today, the standard of care for adult diabetics also includes medications for high blood pressure (usually the ACE inhibitor class of high blood pressure medications), the statin cholesterol medications, and aspirin. It is through these treatments that much of the improvements in the care of type 2 diabetes have taken place.

The primary message for patients with type 2 diabetes is that caution should be used with newer medicines. They are usually very expensive, and as yet, have little proven benefit.

Besides the excessive cost and debatable effects of the newer medications, current debates regarding diabetes care center on optimal blood sugar targets. The hemoglobin A_{1c} (HgbA$_{1c}$) is a test used to gauge blood sugar control in those with diabetes. In the modern era of type 2 diabetes treatment, the goal has been to get the HgbA$_{1c}$ under 7. More recently, it has been recognized that much of the benefits associated with controlling the HgbA$_{1c}$ may occur at much higher levels, even up to 8.5 or 9. In addition, in the past, doctors were encouraged to get the HgbA$_{1c}$ as low as possible. It is now recognized that patients whose HgbA$_{1c}$ is pushed to very low levels may suffer more harm than benefit.

Summary

This is a complicated topic. On the one hand, it is necessary to be cautious about any medical treatment, but not so much that you miss out on the incredible benefits available through the miracles of modern preventive medical care. As they say, don't throw out the baby with the bathwater.

The take-home message is that if you want to maximize the odds that you (and your children) live a long and healthy life, then you should take advantage of the benefits of vaccines and be thankful that we have effective treatments for our most common serious chronic diseases.

Combined with healthy eating and regular exercise, these therapies offer the most reliable and well-researched method we know to lower your risks of developing serious diseases.

Used properly and with appropriate caution, these therapies are remarkably safe. Concerns about the safety of these treatments, while valid, should be balanced against the extremely serious threats posed by the diseases themselves.

The following caveats apply.

Once again, I will emphasize that caution and appropriate monitoring is necessary with all medical treatments.

Side effects from medications do occur. It is usually possible to find a medication, or a combination of medications, that produces few significant side effects. I do not ask my patients to take any long-term medications that make them feel poorly.

Cost and safety are also a significant concern. It is usually possible today to use older generic medications that have proven safety profiles and are substantially more affordable. Caution should be used with any newer medications.

Since I haven't discussed this previously, I will also throw in recommendations here to get appropriate cancer screenings:

- Women ages 21 to 65 should have cervical cancer screening every 3 to 5 years with Pap smears.
- Women should have breast cancer screening with mammograms beginning at age 45 or 50 and every 1 or 2 years (there is controversy surrounding the starting and ending ages for mammograms, as well as the optimal frequency. Discuss this with your clinician).
- Everyone ages 50 to 75 should have colon cancer screening.

In finishing, and in answer to my patient's question, all medicine is not poison. Used properly, and especially when used as part of an overall approach that includes a healthy lifestyle, they are quite the opposite.

PART 3

The *Be Healthy! Workbook*

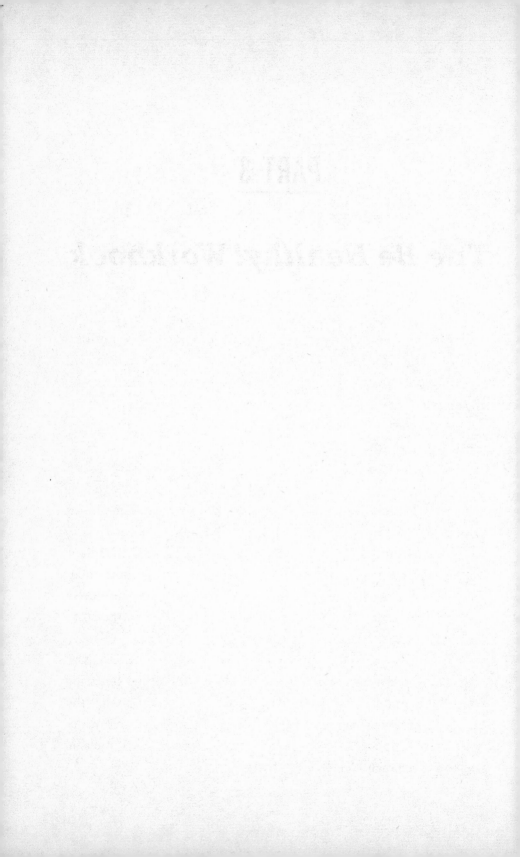

Chapter 1

Introduction to the *Be Healthy! Workbook*

As I hope you remember, the intent of *Staying Alive: The Signs That You Have to See a Doctor Right Now (and the Ways to Avoid Having to See One Again)* is to maximize the odds that you will live a long and healthy life. In the first section, we focused on the importance of receiving medical attention when it is necessary. In the second section, we discussed the miracles of modern preventive medical care.

By far, though (really, really far), the most important way you can improve your overall health-related odds and lower your risks of developing the most serious chronic diseases that affect so many Americans, as well as cancer, is through healthy eating and regular exercise.

In the medical sciences, there is great fanfare when a treatment is able to lower relative risks of becoming ill by more than 10 percent. Doctors and medical researchers become absolutely ecstatic if a treatment shows the potential to lower risks in the 20 to 30 percent range.

Through healthy eating, regular exercise, avoiding tobacco, and controlling your weight, you can lower your risks of serious illness by 80 to 90 percent! In other words, if you want to live a long and healthy life, by far the most important thing you can do is have a healthy lifestyle. There is no medicine, no supplement, no magic bullet available that comes remotely close.

This has been proven in study after study.

In a Swedish study reported in 2014, over 20,000 men were followed for more than ten years. Those who consumed a healthy diet, were physically active, did not smoke, had low levels of abdominal fat, and consumed only moderate amounts of alcohol lowered their risks of having a heart attack by 86 percent!

In another study, whose results were published in the journal *Circulation* in 2012, people who took the best care of themselves through healthy eating, exercise, controlling their weight, and avoidance of smoking lowered their relative risk of death from all causes by 78 percent, and their risk of death from heart disease by 88 percent! These are incredible numbers!

The problem, of course, is that too few of us adhere to what would be considered an optimal lifestyle. That is the reason for the *Be Healthy! Workbook*.

The *Be Healthy! Workbook* is an easy-to-use guided weight loss and health-optimizing system.

The idea underlying the *Be Healthy! Workbook* is to make it as simple as possible to be healthy.

The *Be Healthy! Workbook* offers a simple system to create personalized assignments, goals, and monitoring to improve and then optimize eating and physical fitness habits.

Having trouble controlling your weight? You're not alone. The *Be Healthy! Workbook* provides you with a simple approach to create and maintain the healthy habits needed to control your weight, lose weight, and keep it off.

- Do you overeat or eat portions that are just too large?
- Do you eat too many snacks, junk foods, and sweets?
- Do you eat too much after dinner or eat just before bed?
- Do you have trouble controlling yourself around food?
- Do you eat too much when you are stressed or in a hurry?
- Could you be a food addict?

Again, you are not alone. In fact, most people who have trouble with their weight share many of these common traits. For many people, though, overcoming just one or two of these common issues may hold the secret to being healthy. Many people are intimidated by the thought of having to make huge changes in the way they eat or having to follow all new recipes or meal plans.

The *Be Healthy! Workbook* uses a much easier approach: *identify simple but extremely common eating-related issues and create gradual, easy-to-make changes.* The *Be Healthy! Workbook* has simple strategies to help you identify and overcome your eating-related issues.

Have trouble developing and sticking with an exercise plan? The *Be Healthy! Workbook* will help you *set exercise goals and to stick with those goals.*

The *Be Healthy! Workbook* is designed for anyone and everyone. Whether you have serious weight issues and need to shed pounds, or you are generally fit but want to step it up a notch, this system is for you.

With the *Be Healthy! Workbook*, you will be guided through:

- Unique eating and physical activity assessment tools that identify your specific issues and opportunities for change and improvement
- Transforming your unique issues into specific eating, exercise, and weight loss goals
- Creating monthly eating and fitness assignments
- Monthly monitoring of your progress

The *Be Healthy! Workbook* provides you with a simple yet very flexible approach that takes into account your individual issues and goals. No matter what your beginning eating and fitness status may be, the *Be Healthy! Workbook* gives you the path to improvement.

The *Be Healthy! Workbook* is based on my years of experience as a family physician, talking with patients every day about their weight, eating, and fitness challenges. In those conversations, I hear common themes:

- I hear that most people are plagued by the same easily defined problem eating habits.
  - Oversize portions
  - Eating too many snack foods, junk foods, and sweets
  - Eating too much after dinner or eating meals shortly before bed
  - Drinking too many calorie- and sugar-laden beverages
  - Eating too often at fast-food establishments and restaurants
  - Eating too much bread, pasta, rice, and other refined carbohydrates
  - Compulsive eating, stress eating, and other aspects of food addiction
- I hear most people citing the same barriers that keep them from exercising regularly:
  - Too little time
  - Bad weather
  - Pain
- I hear that most people crave simple solutions because their lives are too busy and the information they receive is too complex.
- I see that when people have the motivation—and when they are given the proper tools—they can be successful!

I have learned that the reason that most people who have been unsuccessful in their quest to lose weight and improve their health fail not because they do not know what to do, and not because they did not find the right diet or exercise regimen. They fail because they don't stick to the plan.

The *Be Healthy! Workbook* is a system to help you stick with it!

Out of daily conversations with my patients, where I hear the same themes over and over, comes a simple solution to help you.

I've developed brief questionnaires that highlight each person's eating and physical activity issues, and by doing so, create a simple strategy for fixing those issues.

The *Be Healthy! Workbook* guides you through this process:

1. Identify your problem eating behaviors and exercise barriers.
2. Create a written plan to systematically eliminate those behaviors and overcome those barriers.
3. Track your progress with monthly calendars.
4. Use frequent assessments to identify your successes and refocus your goals to help overcome challenges that you encounter.

What you need to bring to the table is your motivation. With the proper motivation, you can do anything. The *Be Healthy! Workbook* provides you with a simple, powerful system to make change in your life, but it is your motivation, your desire, and your resolve that are necessary for you to be successful.

The focus of the *Be Healthy! Workbook* is to take you from wherever you are today and progressively and systematically improve your eating and increase the frequency and intensity of your physical activity toward optimal levels. The focus is *not* on one specific weight loss diet, none of which has proven to be superior to another.

The focus is also not on weight loss medication, surgery, or supplements. There is no magic bullet here. However, even if you are interested in trying weight loss medication, surgery, or supplements, and you want to be successful, you will still need to alter your lifestyle, which is the intent of the *Be Healthy! Workbook*.

The focus is on creating and sustaining lifestyle change. The focus is on simplicity. The focus is on creating and sustaining specific healthy eating and exercise habits.

If you have the motivation, the *Be Healthy! Workbook* will help you channel it into action. Because the assignments are only month-long, they are easily digested. Because the goals are specific, they will help you build discipline.

The focus is on *being healthy*—developing and maintaining healthy eating and exercise habits.

Good luck!

Chapter 2

How to Use the
Be Healthy! Workbook

The Quick Guide to Using the *Be Healthy! Workbook*

This guide is for those who want to get going right away. You don't want to do a lot of reading. You are highly motivated, and you want to go! The *Be Healthy! Workbook* will guide you all along the way:

1. Go to Chapter 3, "Motivation," and write down your motivation(s) for change.
2. Then proceed to Chapter 4, "Personal Assessment."
   a. Fill out the **Problem Eating Assessment Tool.**
   b. Fill out the **Physical Activity Assessment Tool.**
3. Next, go to Chapter 5, "Creating Weight, Eating, and Exercise/Fitness Goals."
   a. Write down your **Weight Loss Goals.**
   b. Write down your **Eating Goals.**
   c. Write down your **Physical Activity Goals.**
4. Then, go to Chapter 6, "The Calendars."
   a. Weigh in.
   b. Use your personal **Weight Loss Goals** and **Eating Goals** to create your first month's eating assignment(s).
   c. Based on your personal **Physical Activity Goals,** create your first month's fitness assignment(s).

5. Execute your plan.
   a. Eat less and eat better every day and exercise every day, according to your plan.
   b. Track your daily eating and physical activity achievements on the monthly calendars.
   c. Weigh in regularly.
6. Every 2 to 4 weeks, go to Chapter 7, "Reassessing Progress," to gauge your progress, and if necessary, to create new goals and go again—until you are as nearly perfect as you can be!

The Not-As-Quick Guide to Using the *Be Healthy! Workbook*

There are four steps to achieving optimal health using the *Be Healthy! Workbook:*

1. Assess your current eating and physical activity habits.
2. Determine your motivation for change and set your goals for improved eating and physical activity.
3. Complete monthly eating and physical activity assignments.
4. Complete periodic weigh-ins and assessments.

The *Be Healthy! Workbook* makes things simple.

- Go to Chapter 3, "Motivation," and identify one of the most important determinants of successful change: your personal motivation(s).
- Then go to Chapter 4, "Personal Assessment," and assess your current eating and physical activity habits using:
  - The **Problem Eating Assessment Tool,** a unique method to examine your eating patterns and problems. Each problem you identify also references a corresponding later chapter (the "Assignments"), where you will find detailed information and specific ideas for solutions to your eating issues.

- ○ The **Physical Activity Assessment Tool,** a unique questionnaire that determines where you stand on the exercise spectrum and identifies barriers and opportunities for improvement. Once you complete the questionnaire, you may want to read Chapter 19, "Physical Activity," to learn more about exercise options and how best to plan how you will improve your exercise and physical activity regimens.

- Then, proceed to Chapter 5, "Creating Weight, Eating, and Exercise/Fitness Goals," where you will transform the information you identified in the previous chapters into specific goals and plot your course toward better eating and optimal physical fitness for the next 6 months.

- Proceed to Chapter 6, "The Calendars," where the real work begins.

  - ○ Each month, you will choose your daily eating assignment(s) (you already plotted your assignments in Chapter 5), which you will write down on your **One Month Eating Assignment Calendar.** Initially, your focus will be to eliminate unhealthy eating behaviors, excessive portions, or certain types of foods. Eventually, you will also want to make sure that you are eating as many high-nutrition and nutritionally dense (see "Nutrition 101") foods as possible. Over time, you will optimize your eating and nutrition!

  - ○ In addition, each month you will choose a daily exercise and physical activity goal (from your list in Chapter 5), and you will write it down on your **One Month Exercise and Physical Activity Assignment Calendar.** Each month thereafter, you will increase your exercise frequency, duration, or intensity until you meet your goals. Over time, you will optimize your exercising and physical activity!

  You will track your progress every day on your calendar, indicating those days you successfully achieved your goal(s).

  You will weigh yourself regularly, at least once per week (some people find it useful to weigh themselves every day), and record the results on your calendar.

- In Chapter 7, "Reassessing Progress," you will assess your progress every 2 to 4 weeks. If you are achieving your goals, you can continue as planned. If you are not, you may need to reaffirm your commitment or make changes that will help you be more successful. If necessary or helpful, you might even choose to repeat assignments that were especially hard or important for you.

Chapters 8 through 19 contain helpful information to directly support the work you are doing in the *Be Healthy! Workbook*. Chapters 8, 9, and 10 provide valuable information that will help you along your path to change and health optimization.

- Chapter 8, "On Being Healthy," discusses the aspects of a healthy life, with an emphasis, of course, on the need for healthy eating *and* daily physical activity.
- Chapter 9, "Losing Weight," reviews the most recent developments in weight loss science and provides useful and up-to-date information and specific approaches regarding what works best for successful weight loss and weight control.
- Chapter 10, "Nutrition 101," summarizes and simplifies what we know today about nutrition; it also sorts out much of the controversy and confusion regarding nutrition and weight control.

Chapters 11 through 18 are a menu of eating-related assignments. Each chapter corresponds directly to one of the issues listed in the eating assessment tool and provides helpful information that will help you to create your monthly plans and assignments.

- Chapter 11, "Controlling Eating Behavior," and Chapter 12, "Portion Control," are mandatory assignments because so many of us struggle with these issues, and mastering them is central to successful weight loss and weight control. You can choose at which point you want to do these two assignments. They can be challenging issues, and you may want to choose an easier assignment early on just to get your feet wet. But if portion control and uncontrolled eating behavior are your biggest issues, you may want to start with those!

- Chapter 13, "Cutting Snacks, Sweets, and Junk Foods," will be useful for the many people whose weight control issues relate to excessive snacking, sweet eating, and junk foods.

- Chapter 14, "Stopping Night Eating," is for the many people who eat too much food in the evening, late at night, and after dinner.

- Chapter 15, "Cutting Beverage Sugar and Calories," will help those people who get their extra calories by drinking sugary, high-calorie beverages.

- Chapter 16, "Fast Food and Restaurant Eating," focuses on those of us who eat out at restaurants and fast-food establishments, where it is so easy to overeat and so hard to get proper nutrition.

- Chapter 17, "Reducing White Breads, Pastas, and Refined Carbs," will be a help to those of us who eat too much bread, pastas, and other foods made from refined carbohydrates, which we now know may pack on the pounds and increase our risks of heart and cardiovascular disease.

- Chapter 18, "Optimal Nutrition," provides simple methods to optimize your eating, adding the vegetables and fruit that are the cornerstone of good nutrition.

- Chapter 19, "Physical Activity," reviews the most recent recommendations for physical activity and contains many tips that will help you optimize your exercise and physical activity habits.

Chapter 3

Motivation

Your motivation to make change is where the process must begin. *The number one determinant* of your success in improving your health, in making significant changes in your life, and in losing weight is your *motivation*.

Study after study shows this to be true. My experience, day in and day out with patients, shows this to be true. People who have the motivation to change can achieve extraordinary results.

I find that a person's motivation is the key to successfully navigating two important moments:

- Getting started. You must have a compelling reason to want to begin to make significant, often difficult changes in your life.
- When you experience a bump in the road or even failure, strong, clear motivation is often the only thing that helps you persevere when the going gets tough.

You must have the motivation to make significant changes in your life. You must expect and be ready to deal with the numerous barriers you will experience, as well as the very real possibility of temporary setbacks, and even the possibility of failure, in order to achieve true lasting change. With the proper motivation, it can be done!

Here are some of the common concepts that people tell me motivate them to make change:

- **Weight loss.** Many people want to lose weight! This goal provides strong motivation to many people.
- **To look and feel better.** Many people tell me they just want to look and feel better. That is legitimate motivation, especially if you are vain (like me!).
- **To be physically capable to help family or other loved ones in need.** Many people I speak with want to ensure that they can be there for a family member, help a spouse or parent, or provide for and be present for their children or grandchildren. That is excellent motivation!
- **To alleviate or prevent pain.** Many people who are overweight develop pain issues. The best way to treat that pain is to lose weight and strengthen joints and muscles. To decrease pain is fantastic motivation!
- **Being able to continue to do the things you enjoy.** The number one sign that my patients are beginning to age is when they tell me that they can no longer do the things they liked to do. They can't go shopping. They can no longer travel. This indicates to me that they have lost muscle strength. I see patients who appear old at the age of 50 and those who appear young at 80. What determines the difference? Muscle strength and weight control make the biggest difference! Being able to continue doing the things you enjoy is great motivation!
- **To live a long and joyful life.** If you think about it, what we want most is a long and joyful life. Isn't that true? The best thing we can do to ensure a long and joyful life is to preserve our health. Wanting to live a long and joy-filled life may be your motivation.

As an exercise, spend some time thinking about your life and health goals, and what motivates you to make real change in your life. Then, in the space below, write down some (or all) of those things. What you write down will be used every month as a reminder, a tool to help you stay your course to being and staying healthy.

My Motivation(s) to Make Change and Be Healthy

1. _____
2. _____
3. _____
4. _____
5. _____
6. _____
7. _____
8. _____
9. _____
10. _____

Chapter 4

Personal Assessment

The next step in your journey toward optimal health is to assess your current status. This step will enable you to plot your course for the future.

The **Problem Eating Assessment Tool** is the crux of the *Be Healthy! Workbook*'s simple but systematic approach to improving your eating and controlling your weight.

The **Physical Activity Assessment Tool** provides a simple yet powerful method to gauge your current exercise and physical activity status (or lack thereof) and the issues that keep you from exercising more.

Then, in Chapter 5, "Creating Weight, Eating, and Exercise/ Fitness Goals," your answers will be used to create your personal plan for achieving optimal eating, an optimal physical activity regimen for life, and your personal weight loss goals.

So take some time to fill out both the **Problem Eating Assessment Tool** and the **Physical Activity Assessment Tool.** The more detail you include, the more thought you give your answers, the more material you will have with which to form your plan for changing and optimizing your lifestyle patterns.

Problem Eating Assessment Tool

Name: _____ Date: _____

Place a check in the box next to any of the following items that characterize your current eating patterns. Then, in the space provided, describe your issues in more detail. Include the specific type(s) of problem foods that you eat, the amounts you eat, the times you eat these foods, and any other information you feel might be pertinent.

☐ I just eat too much: I eat too much food, I eat too often, and/ or I eat portions that are too large (see Chapter 11, "Controlling Eating Behavior," and Chapter 12, "Portion Control," for help with these issues).
Details: _____
_____

☐ I eat too many sweets and snack/junk foods (see Chapter 13, "Cutting Snacks, Sweets, and Junk Foods," for help with this issue).
Details: _____
_____

☐ I snack too much at night or after dinner (see Chapter 14, "Stopping Night Eating," and Chapter 11, "Controlling Eating Behavior," for help with these issues).
Details: _____
_____

☐ I drink too many beverages that have sugar or calories (soda, juice, sweet tea, milk, alcohol) (see Chapter 15, "Cutting Beverage Sugar and Calories," for help with this issue).
Details: _____
_____

☐ I tend to eat meals late in the evening or right before going to bed (see Chapter 14, "Stopping Night Eating," and Chapter 11, "Controlling Eating Behavior," for help with these issues).
Details: _____
_____

☐ I eat fast foods too often or eat at restaurants for too many of my meals (see Chapter 16, "Fast Food and Restaurant Eating," and Chapter 11, "Controlling Eating Behavior," for help with these issues).
Details: _____

_____

☐ I eat a lot of bread and refined carbohydrates (white breads and pastas) (see Chapter 17, "Reducing White Breads, Pastas, and Refined Carbs," for help with this issue).
Details: _____

_____

☐ I eat too quickly, and tend to eat large amounts of food in a short amount of time (see Chapter 11, "Controlling Eating Behavior," and Chapter 12, "Portion Control," for help with these issues).
Details: _____

_____

☐ I am a compulsive eater and tend to eat when I am stressed, unhappy, or for other reasons besides being hungry (see Chapter 11, "Controlling Eating Behavior," for help with this issue).
Details: _____

_____

☐ I have trouble controlling myself around food. I am a food addict (see Chapter 11, "Controlling Eating Behavior," for help with this issue).
Details: _____

_____

☐ I skip breakfast (see Chapter 9, "Losing Weight," for information on why skipping breakfast may make it hard for you to lose weight).
Details: _____

_____

☐ I don't eat enough healthy foods (vegetables, salads, fruits, beans) (see Chapter 18, "Optimal Nutrition," for help with this issue.
Details: _____

_____

Other issues:

_____

_____

_____

Physical Activity Assessment Tool

Name: _____ Date: _____

You may want to read Chapter 19, "Physical Activity," which reviews the most recent recommendations for physical activity and contains many tips that will help you to optimize your exercise and physical activity habits.

As you are filling out the **Physical Activity Assessment Tool,** keep in mind:

- The ultimate goal is to exercise at least 30 to 60 minutes per day at a moderate to vigorous level of intensity (or the highest level of intensity you are capable of), with strength training on at least 2 days per week.
- You will need to create a plan to get from where you are currently, in terms of exercise duration and level of intensity, to your goal.

Place a check in the box next to the following items that best characterize your physical activity patterns, and then, where appropriate, briefly describe your issues in more detail.

Current Exercise Frequency

☐ I do not exercise regularly or get any physical activity on a regular basis.

☐ I do exercise, but sporadically or not regularly enough.
  If you checked this item, please fill in the information below.

- How many days per week do you exercise, on average?

  _____

- How many minutes per day do you exercise, on average?

  _____

- What type(s) of exercise do you engage in most of the time?

  _____

☐ I do exercise regularly, but I could exercise more frequently or for a longer time.
  If you checked this item, please fill in the information below.

- How many days per week do you exercise, on average?

  _____

- How many minutes per day do you exercise, on average?

  _____

- What type(s) of exercise do you engage in most of the time?

  _____

Current Exercise Intensity Level

☐ I think that I currently exercise at the highest level of intensity that I am capable of.

If you checked this item, please fill in the information below.

How would you rate the intensity of your current physical activities (you can see Chapter 19, "Physical Activity," which defines moderate and vigorous intensity exercise)?

☐ Light
☐ Moderate
☐ Vigorous

Other Pertinent Details:

_____

_____

_____

_____

☐ I think I am capable of exercising at a higher level of intensity (at least some of the time).

If you checked this item, please fill in the information below.

How would you rate the intensity of your current physical activities (you can see Chapter 19, "Physical Activity," which defines moderate and vigorous intensity exercise)?

☐ Light
☐ Moderate
☐ Vigorous

Other Pertinent Details:

_____

_____

_____

_____

Types of Exercise You Currently Engage In

☐ When I exercise, I tend to focus only on cardiovascular fitness (walking, jogging, running, biking, aerobics).
If you checked this item, please fill in the information below.
What type(s) of exercise do you engage in most of the time?

_____

Is there any form of strength training that you would be interested in trying?

_____

_____

☐ When I exercise, I tend to focus only on strength training.
If you checked this item, please fill in the information below.
What type(s) of exercise do you engage in most of the time?

_____

Is there any form of cardiovascular training that you would be interested in trying?

_____

_____

Barriers to Exercise

☐ I tend not to exercise when the weather is bad or it is too hot or too cold.
If you checked this item, please fill in the information below.
What options for exercise do you have if the weather is not good for outdoor activity?

☐ Home equipment: _____

☐ Home video workouts: _____

☐ Gym: _____

☐ Fitness classes: _____

☐ Other: _____

☐ I tend not to exercise, or I miss workouts, because of schedule constraints.

If you checked this item, please use the following space to detail the specific aspects of your schedule, days of the week, or times of day when you find it more difficult to exercise.

_____

_____

_____

☐ I tend not to exercise because of pain-related issues or other physical health problems.

If you checked this item, please fill in the information below.

Do you have access to any of the following types of exercise that tend to be better tolerated by people with knee, hip, and ankle or foot pain issues?

    ☐ Elliptical machine

    ☐ Recumbent stationary bike

    ☐ Treadmill

    ☐ Swimming pool

    ☐ Pool aerobics

    ☐ Tai chi

    ☐ Pilates

☐ I do not exercise enough because I find it boring and lose interest.

If you checked this item, please fill in the information below.

What type(s) of physical activity did you enjoy when you were younger?

_____

_____

_____

Is there any type of physical activity that you have been interested in trying?

_____

_____

Other Notes/Comments/Ideas

_____

_____

_____

_____

Chapter 5

Creating Weight, Eating, and Exercise/Fitness Goals

One of the keys to making successful change is to have a *concrete, written plan*. In this section, we use the information you identified in the preceding Chapter 4 with the **Problem Eating Assessment Tool** and the **Physical Activity Assessment Tool,** and transform that information into specific eating and exercise goals.

Those eating and exercise goals will then be used to create a written plan to lose weight, improve your eating, and to optimize your physical activity regimen! Then, in the next chapter, you will execute your plan, with the help of our monthly calendars.

Remember that the ultimate goal is to go from where you are currently on the eating and exercise spectrum and to optimize your eating and exercise patterns. But first, you need to know where you are headed. As a first exercise, write down your personal weight loss goals.

Weight Loss Goals

Date: _____

Starting Weight: _____

Goal Weight: _____

Monthly Weight Loss Goal: _____

Total Weight Loss Goal: _____

Next, you will create your personal *eating* optimization plan, and then your *exercise* optimization plan.

Creating Your Eating Goals

This is straightforward. Go to Chapter 4, "Personal Assessment," and review your **Problem Eating Assessment Tool.**

Each eating-related issue that you identified with a check will now be turned around to become one of your eating goals. For instance, if you identified snacking and sweet eating as one of your issues, then one of your eating goals will be to eliminate or reduce your snacking and sweet eating. Simple, isn't it?

If you identified snacking after dinner as one of your problem eating habits, then it makes sense that one of your eating goals will be to eliminate after-dinner snacking.

Each problem eating habit that you eliminate also removes a significant corresponding number of calories. Systematically eliminating your problem eating habits (in addition to increasing exercise), therefore, also becomes your systematic plan for weight loss.

The collection of problem eating habits that you identify and the corresponding solutions and goals each item creates, becomes a simple, concrete plan to optimize your eating and help you lose weight. Here is an example of the two-step process at work.

Step 1: Use the issues identified in the **Problem Eating Assessment Tool** to create your eating goals.

Eating Issue (from Chapter 4)	How I Will Solve the Issue
I just eat too much: I eat too much food, too often, and portions that are too large.	I will eat smaller portions by eating lunch and dinner on smaller plates.
I eat too many sweets and snack/ junk foods.	I will eliminate sweets (except for one per week).

I snack too much at night or after dinner.	I will stop eating at 7:00 p.m. I will use the "12-hour window" plan, and eat only between 7:00 a.m. and 7:00 p.m.
I drink too many beverages that have sugar or calories.	I will eliminate all beverages that have calories. I will drink only water.
I eat too quickly and tend to eat large amounts of food in a short amount of time.	I will slow down my eating. I will relax prior to eating by breathing deeply for 60 seconds prior to every meal. I will take a deep breath between every mouthful of food.
I don't eat enough healthy foods.	I will eat at least 7 servings of vegetables and fruit per day by having a salad at lunch every day, having a serving of fruit with each meal, and changing all my snacks to berries, apples, or bananas.

Next, decide how you will time the changes you will make and create your written plan. First, think about the following questions:

1. Do you prefer to set small, attainable goals as you work toward a higher goal?
   If the answer is yes, you can choose to implement your plan gradually over time, adding a new eating goal each month.
2. Do you prefer to try and achieve the highest, most aggressive goals right away?
   If this sounds more like your style, then create your goals to reflect that.

Or you may choose to make a few changes at one time. Choose whichever approach feels right for you.

Step 2: Use what you wrote in the Step 1 table ("How I Will Solve the Issue") to create a written schedule to optimize your eating.

Eating Goals/Plan

Time	Eating Goal
Month 1	I will eat smaller portions by eating lunch and dinner on smaller plates.
Month 2	I will eliminate sweets (except for one per week).
Month 3	I will stop eating at 7:00 p.m. I will use the "12-hour window" plan, and eat only between 7:00 a.m. and 7:00 p.m.
Month 4	I will eliminate all beverages that have calories. I will drink only water.
Month 5	I will slow down my eating. I will relax prior to eating by breathing deeply for 60 seconds prior to every meal. I will take a deep breath between every mouthful of food.
Month 6	I will eat at least 7 servings of vegetables and fruit per day by having a salad at lunch every day, having a serving of fruit with each meal, and changing all my snacks to berries, apples, or bananas.

Now it is your turn. In the table below, write each of the eating issues identified in Chapter 4 (on the left), and then generate specific written solutions to each of the issues (on the right).

Step 1: Use the issues identified in the **Problem Eating Assessment Tool** to create your eating goals.

Eating Issue (from Chapter 4)	How I Will Solve the Issue

Step 2: Use what you wrote in the Step 1 table ("How I Will Solve the Issue" to create a written schedule to optimize your eating.

Eating Goals/Plan

Time	Eating Goal

Creating Your Physical Activity Goals

Creating your physical activity goals and plan is simple as well.

- Remember: the ultimate goal is to exercise at least 30 to 60 minutes per day at a moderate to vigorous level of intensity (or the highest level of intensity you are capable of), and to include strength training on at least 2 days per week.
- You need to create a plan to get from where you are currently, in terms of exercise duration and level of intensity, to your goal.

A few caveats:

- If you want to exercise more than the goal stated above, and you enjoy doing more, then do more!
- If you are unable to exercise at a moderate or vigorous level of intensity, then you should not. *Do your best to exercise at whatever level you are capable of.* Of course, it is important to note that you should consult your physician prior to the start of an exercise program.

To create your physical activity goals and plan, first go again to Chapter 4 and consult your **Physical Activity Assessment Tool.** Each exercise-related issue that you identified with a check will now be turned around to become one of your exercise goals.

For instance, if one of your issues is "I do exercise, but sporadically or not regularly enough," then you will create a plan to gradually increase your exercise frequency to every day.

If one of your issues is "I think I am capable of exercising at a higher level of intensity (at least some of the time)," you will create a plan to increase the intensity level of your current fitness activities, for instance, by taking a Zumba class or adding some high-intensity interval training (HIIT) workouts.

The collection of exercise issues that you identified, and the corresponding solutions and goals each item creates, becomes a simple, concrete plan to optimize your exercise regimen.

Remember, ultimately you want your plan to get you to the point that you exercise at least 30 to 60 minutes per day at a moderate to vigorous level of intensity (or the highest level of intensity you are capable of), and to include strength training on at least two days per week.

Here is an example of the two-step process at work. There are other sample plans that you may refer to, or even use as your own, in an appendix at the end of the book.

Let's say that you currently exercise two or three times per week, going to the gym and using a treadmill for 30 minutes of comfortable walking. In addition, you decide that your goal is to exercise 30 minutes per day at a vigorous level of intensity. You want to reach your goal in 6 months.

Step 1: Use the issues identified in the **Physical Activity Assessment Tool** to create your physical activity goals.

Current Physical Activity Assessment/Issues	Optimal Physical Activity Plan/Solutions
I do exercise, but sporadically or not regularly enough.	I will start at 5 days per week in Month 1. I will increase to 7 days per week in Month 2. Eventually, when I am in better shape, I would like to try P90X. (P90X is a well-known video-based workout system developed by the popular fitness instructor, Tony Horton, and sold by Beachbody.com.)
I think I am capable of exercising at a higher level of intensity (at least some of the time).	I will increase intensity by replacing some of my walking with Zumba workouts. I will add intensity to my walking workouts by working in 10-minute HIIT workouts (see Chapter 19, "Physical Activity"). Eventually, I want to try the P90X workouts.

When I exercise, I tend to focus only on cardiovascular fitness.	Starting in Month 2, I will do workouts with a strength-training focus at least 2 days per week.
I tend not to exercise when the weather is bad or it is too hot or too cold.	I will walk outside when the weather is nice but will use my treadmill or an exercise DVD when the weather is uncooperative.
I tend not to exercise, or I miss workouts, because of schedule constraints.	On days that I know I will be working later, I will schedule my workout in the morning. For days that my schedule prevents going to the gym or the track, I will use my 30-minute PiYo (PiYo is a series video-based workouts developed by Chalene Johnson and marketed by Beachbody.com) workout DVD at home.

Next, decide on how you will time the changes you will make, and create your written plan.

Step 2: Use the **Optimal Physical Activity Plan/Solutions** from Step 1 to create a written schedule to optimize your Physical Activity regimen.

Time	Physical Activity Goals
Month 1	Increase to 5 days per week of comfortable walking 30 minutes per day at the Rail Trail, right after work. On Tuesdays, because I usually work later, I will walk in the morning. If the weather is bad, I will walk at home on the treadmill.

Time	Physical Activity Goals
Month 2	Walk 5 days per week at a moderate-intensity level and add two light strength-training workouts per week, Thursday night and Saturdays. On Tuesdays, because I usually work later, I will walk in the morning. If the weather is bad, I will walk at home on the treadmill.
Month 3	Begin taking one-hour Zumba class on Monday and Wednesday evenings at the gym. On Tuesdays, Thursdays, Saturdays, walk 30 minutes per day at moderate intensity (if the weather is bad, I will walk at home on the treadmill). On Fridays and Sundays, I will do strength-training workouts at the gym.
Month 4	Continue one-hour Zumba class on Monday and Wednesday evenings at the gym. On Tuesdays, Thursdays, Saturdays, walk 20 minutes per day at moderate intensity, and end with a 10-minute HIIT workout (see Chapter 19, "Physical Activity"). If the weather is bad, I will walk at home on the treadmill. On Fridays and Sundays, I will do strength-training workouts at the gym.
Month 5	Continue Zumba 2 days per week; for 3 days per week, do two 10-minute HIIT workouts separated by 10 minutes of moderate-intensity walking; 2 days per week of strength training (increasing intensity).
Month 6	Begin P90X3 program, 6 days per week. Jog lightly for 30 minutes on off day.

Now it is your turn. In the table below, write each of the physical activity issues identified in Chapter 4 on the left, and then generate specific written solutions to each of the issues on the right.

Step 1: Use the issues identified in the **Physical Activity Assessment Tool** to create your physical activity goals.

Current Physical Activity Assessment/Issues	Optimal Physical Activity Goals/ Solutions

Next, decide on how you will time the changes you will make and create your written plan.

Step 2: Use the **Optimal Physical Activity Plan/Solutions** from Step 1 to create a written schedule to optimize your Physical Activity regimen.

Time	Physical Activity Goals

Note

Think of the plans you created as a starting point or the first point on a map. The plan you made today is not set in stone.

As you go along, you will want to revisit your goals and plans, which may change based on your successes (or failures). You may find one of your goals especially challenging and choose to repeat it the next month, and even the month after that.

Your written goals and plans are a living document. Use the given forms as a model to create new ones as needed.

Chapter 6

The Calendars

This is where things get serious. The following pages contain your one-month eating and one-month physical activity assignment calendars. Fill them out and create new ones as needed using these samples. This is where the real change will take place.

At the beginning of each month, you will write out on your calendar your one-month eating and physical activity goals, which you will take directly from the plan you created in Chapter 5.

Your plan now comes to life! Each day that you are successful in achieving your goal(s), check that day's box. There is also space to make notes, if that is helpful. Record your weight at least once per week but more often if you feel it is helpful.

Enjoy Being Healthy!

One-Month Eating Assignment Calendar

Name:_____ Date:_____

Nutrition Goal(s):

_____

_____

Motivation:_____

Starting Weight: _____ lbs.

Weight Loss Goal for the Month: _____ lbs.

Sunday	Monday	Tuesday	Wednesday	Thursday	Friday	Saturday
Success___ Weight___	Success___	Success___	Success___	Success___	Success___	Success___
Success___ Weight___	Success___	Success___	Success___	Success___	Success___	Success___
Success___ Weight___	Success___	Success___	Success___	Success___	Success___	Success___
Success___ Weight___	Success___	Success___	Success___	Success___	Success___	Success___
Success___ Weight___	Success___	Success___	Success___	Success___	Success___	Success___

One-Month Exercise and Physical Activity Assignment Calendar

Physical Activity Goal(s):_____

Sunday	Monday	Tuesday	Wednesday	Thursday	Friday	Saturday
Success___	Success___	Success___	Success___	Success___	Success___	Success___
Success___	Success___	Success___	Success___	Success___	Success___	Success___
Success___	Success___	Success___	Success___	Success___	Success___	Success___
Success___	Success___	Success___	Success___	Success___	Success___	Success___
Success___	Success___	Success___	Success___	Success___	Success___	Success___

Ending Weight:_____ lbs.

Chapter 7

Reassessing Progress

Assessing how you are doing is a process you will want to go through every 2 to 4 weeks, depending on your preferences and how you feel you are doing in your quest to achieve optimal health.

A brief note about success and failure: many of us feel disappointment if we do not attain our goals, or if we experience setbacks and challenges. But setbacks, challenges, and even failure (temporary failure) are just part of the process that may be necessary for us to attain success. They should be expected when we are trying to accomplish something of value.

- Don't give up!
- Learn something, at least one thing, from each setback, challenge, or failure.
- Always ask yourself how you could do things differently or better.
- Make something good come from each setback, challenge, or failure.

Remember,

- You can repeat assignments that were especially helpful.
- If your results are not satisfactory to you, you may want to read (or reread) the chapter that pertains to your eating or physical activity assignment for more ideas.
- If you were having success and then stop making progress, be ready to make changes.

- Be ready for hard work, especially at first. With time, things should get easier.

Please answer the following questions and follow the outlined pathway:

1. Are you successfully achieving your eating, exercise, and weight loss goals?
    a. **No**: Go to **Number 2.**
    b. **Yes**: Congratulations! Continue with your current plans. Answer this question: what has been the key to your success so far?

    _____

2. Don't give up! Don't stop! Remember your motivation(s) (see Chapter 3). You can do this! Go to **Number 3.**
3. Check the box(es) that best characterize your experience:
    ☐ Unsuccessful at attaining your *eating goals*.
       Answer the following questions:
       1. What do you think the problem is?

           _____

       2. What is the key to doing better?

           _____

       3. How can you do things better?

           _____

       Go to **Number 4.**
    ☐ Unsuccessful at attaining your *exercise goals*.
       Answer the following questions:
       1. What do you this the problem is?

           _____

       2. What is the key to doing better?

           _____

       3. How can you do things better?

           _____

       Go to **Number 4.**

☐   Successfully attained your eating and exercise goals but did
not lose weight. Go to **Number 5**.

4. If you did not attain your eating and/or exercise goals, you have
two choices:

a.   Try again using the same goals. You could have done better
with the goals you already created. Create another calendar,
using the same goals. You can do this!

b.   Rework your goals and plans.

5. You will need to create more aggressive eating and/or exercise
goals. You have three choices:

a.   Rework your *eating goals and plans* only.

b.   Rework your *exercise goals and plans* only.

c.   Rework both your *eating and exercise goals and plans*.

Chapter 8

On Being Healthy

Being healthy can mean a lot of things. To me, being healthy means doing the best we can to take care of the bodies we are given. Being healthy doesn't guarantee that you won't become ill, but it improves the chances that you will stay well. At any point along the wellness/illness spectrum, we can do our best to be healthy and to improve our health.

Being healthy is simple. To be healthy, we need to:

- Eat healthy.
- Be physically active.
- Avoid tobacco.
- Avoid excessive alcohol.
- Get adequate sleep.

That is a short list because I think it is important to keep it simple.

Admittedly, this list focuses on physical health, but we should not ignore the mind or the spirit. That is a different topic, though, and not the focus of this workbook. I *will* say here that we all need to learn to deal with stress (notice that I didn't say avoid stress).

I focus on physical health because it is the aspect of our health over which we have the most direct control and because improving our physical health has such obvious benefits.

Need proof? To prove this point, let's take a morbid look at life. Every year, the US government (Centers for Disease Control and Prevention [CDC], National Center for Health Statistics [NCHS]) tallies up the most common causes of death. For the year 2011, they were as follows:

- Heart disease: 596,577
- Cancer: 576,691
- Chronic lower respiratory diseases: 142,943
- Stroke (cerebrovascular diseases): 128,932
- Accidents (unintentional injuries): 126,438
- Alzheimer's disease: 84,974
- Diabetes: 73,831
- Influenza and pneumonia: 53,826
- Nephritis, nephrotic syndrome, and nephrosis: 45,591
- Intentional self-harm (suicide): 39,518

A quick analysis of this list leads me to the conclusion that the secret to long life and good health is being healthy (as defined above).

The majority of the conditions listed above *can be prevented* to a significant extent. The risk factors for developing heart disease (our nation's number one killer), stroke, Alzheimer's disease, and diabetes are nearly the same:

- Family history
- Obesity
- Unhealthy eating
- Sedentary lifestyle (lack of physical activity)
- Smoking tobacco

The top risk factors for developing cancer include some of the same:

- Increasing age
- Tobacco use
- Obesity

The number one risk factor for developing "chronic lower respiratory disease" (emphysema, chronic obstructive pulmonary disease [COPD], asthma) is smoking, of course.

We see a repeating theme, don't we? Of course we do!

Added to that, studies demonstrate that a healthy lifestyle can prevent 85 to 90 percent of heart disease, stroke, and diabetes, almost all cases of emphysema and COPD (which relates to smoking), and a significant number of cases of cancer and Alzheimer's disease.

Add to that relatively new data that suggest that the biggest overall risk to life and limb is *sitting*! Being sedentary—on the couch, at work, in front of the computer, or in front of the TV—kills!

So, the secret to long life and good health is clear:

- Eat healthy.
- Exercise regularly.
- Don't smoke.

It is also interesting to look at the costs of health care in the United States. Two-thirds of every dollar spent on health care in the United States goes toward preventable chronic diseases (in other words, heart disease, stroke, diabetes, COPD). Two-thirds!

What is the number one problem with the American health-care system? It is by far the costliest health-care system in the world.

But if two-thirds of health-care expenses go toward preventable chronic diseases, and 85 percent of preventable chronic diseases are *preventable* (through healthy eating, exercise, and avoiding tobacco) . . . then we could fix the number one problem of the American health-care system . . . *by being healthy!*

Feeling patriotic? Be healthy!

Chapter 9

Losing Weight

In this section, you will learn about the latest research and techniques to help you create a successful weight control and weight loss plan.

The Math of Weight Loss

- If your weight is stable, your energy intake *matches* your body's energy demands.
- If you are gaining weight, your energy intake *exceeds* your body's energy demands.

If you want to lose weight, your energy intake must be less than your body's energy demands. To lose weight, therefore, we can either decrease our energy intake (decrease calories that we consume) or increase our body's energy demands (burn more calories).

How much of a calorie deficit do we need to create to lose weight? The answer is somewhat controversial, but there is a simple way to clear up the controversy. The traditional rule of thumb is that a pound of fat equals 3,500 calories. If that is true, then all we need to do to lose a pound of body fat is to combine reduced calorie intake and increased energy demands (physical activity) to the tune of 3,500 calories.

The problem is that this equation frequently doesn't hold true in the real world. Our body's energy metabolism is more complicated than that. But that doesn't mean that we need to make weight loss complicated. It can still be simple.

The answer is that to lose weight, you need to take in fewer calories than you *currently* take in, to burn off more calories than you *currently* burn, or both.

The answer to how many calories you need to cut or burn to lose weight is in your scale and in your mirror (my wife says, "It's also in how your jeans fit.").

When trying to lose weight, you need to:

1. Create a strategy to eat less food (or possibly different foods) *than you currently eat.*
2. Create a strategy to exercise more frequently, for a longer period of time, or at a higher intensity level *than you currently do.*
3. Choose a weight loss goal (short and long term).
4. Execute your plan successfully.
5. Monitor your weight and look in the mirror (or pay attention to how your jeans feel).
6. If your scale and mirror tell you that you are losing weight, then you have chosen the proper combination of calorie reduction and increased physical activity.
7. If your scale and mirror tell you that you are not losing weight (or you were losing weight, but then you stop), adjust your strategy.

The reason that you need to look at both your scale *and* your mirror is that weight can sometimes be deceiving. If you begin to exercise in a manner that increases muscle mass, then it is possible that you could gain weight but still change your body in a positive way.

On the other hand, many of us look in the mirror and see something other than reality: we look heavier or even lighter to ourselves than we do to others. So the mirror isn't always an accurate measure, either. That is why you need to look at both the scale *and* the mirror.

In addition, what works successfully for a period of time may not continue to work if the body's metabolism changes, or it may not continue to provide the same results. Our bodies' energy demands may change as our weight, food intake, or physical activity changes. That is why we suggest that if your weight loss strategy was once resulting in weight loss, and then the weight loss stops, then your strategy needs to be adjusted.

To summarize, if you want to lose weight, eat less than you currently eat, exercise more than you currently exercise, or both, and monitor your progress. That's simple!

Do Certain Foods Promote Weight Loss More Than Others?

This is an intriguing question, isn't it? Maybe we gain weight or have difficulty losing weight because we are eating the wrong foods. Maybe we can lose weight merely by changing the content of our diet, rather than the amount of food we eat, and can avoid having to go hungry when trying to lose weight. Maybe we can choose foods that satisfy our hunger better than others and reduce pounds without having to feel hungry.

And maybe, just maybe, there is a food that is the magic bullet, a food that we can eat that will lead to weight loss! Wouldn't that be great?

Those are the questions we all wonder about when it comes to diet and weight:

1. Are there foods that encourage weight loss more than others?
2. Are there foods that encourage weight gain more than others?
3. Are there foods that will satisfy our hunger better than others?
4. Can we lose weight without having to work at it?

The answer to questions 1 through 3 is: maybe, maybe not! Sorry, but that's the answer. The answer to question 4 is: probably not.

In the 1980s and 1990s, we were told that if we wanted to lose weight we should eat lots of foods that contain carbohydrates, "carbs." Carbs have only 4 calories per gram (compared to fat, which has 9 calories per gram), and therefore if we fill up on carbs, we should lose weight because our diet tends to be lower in calories. And yet, despite an emphasis on added dietary carbs, people's weights began to climb.

Then along came Dr. Atkins, who recommended the exact opposite approach. He suggested that eating fat and protein would lead to more weight loss and even better health. And the foods you were supposed to eat, according to Dr. Atkins, were the fun foods—like bacon! Amazing success stories (and great marketing) abounded.

But then, lots of the people who had lost so much weight with the Atkins approach began to gain their weight back. There were even indications that the Atkins approach might be a risky way to eat, possibly increasing the risk of heart attack and stroke.

Since then, there has been no shortage of weight loss books, fads, and other new approaches. Is one better than another?

The current answer is: probably not. In what appears to be the most definitive study comparing weight loss results using high-carb versus low-carb approaches, weight loss results were relatively similar. What determined the amount of weight loss more than anything else was not the content of the food, but how well someone adhered to the diet.

Is the question entirely settled? Not yet.

Probably the most interesting research to date regarding food choices, hunger, and appetite is the work of Barbara Rolls, PhD, whose work is detailed in her excellent book *Volumetrics*. She suggests that people tend to eat the same volume of food every day, and that you can lower the calorie content of what you eat by adding liquid to the foods you consume.

Anecdotally, many people tell me that high-protein meals tend to satisfy their hunger better than high-carb meals. My own experience is that there is nothing like a banana to control my hunger between meals. You may need to experiment to find out what works best for you.

There are also recent studies that suggest that lower-carb approaches to eating may be better at controlling blood sugar in people with diabetes, and that diets high in refined carbs and sugars may have negative effects on our health and our weight. There are even some studies suggesting that sugar substitutes, at very high doses, may fool the body (the body thinks it is real sugar) and encourage weight gain.

For now, the focus should be on *adherence*. Whatever eating approach you feel aligns best with your eating preferences is probably best for you, but you must stick with it!

Do You Need to Go Hungry?

Many diets tout their ability to create weight loss without hunger. The idea is appealing and important, because we are more likely to stick with a diet if it does not cause pangs of hunger for too long of a time. But do we need to feel hungry to lose weight?

I think the answer is yes—at least for a short time. When many of us *first* make significant changes in how we eat (eating less, that is), our bodies often fight back against the change. The sensations we feel, be it actual hunger or just the anxiety we feel when we think we are hungry, are part of a complicated effort our bodies make to keep us from making those changes. That is the complicated nature of hunger and appetite, food-related behaviors, and food addictions.

When we cut back on eating, or significantly change the way we eat, our body (and our mind) tries to convince us not to do it. That is because many of us are addicted to food and to how we eat. In other words, many of us are food and eating addicts.

I believe that one of the reasons that we have so much trouble losing weight is that we have failed to recognize the prevalence and impact of food addictions. Think about it.

- Do you have a pattern of difficulty controlling yourself around food?
- Do you feel the urge to eat when you know you shouldn't be hungry?
- Do you frequently end up eating more than you had planned to eat?
- Do you feel hungry shortly after you have just finished a meal?
- Do you eat compulsively throughout the day?
- Do you find it hard to stop eating even when you are full?
- Do you binge and feel bad about it afterwards?

You are not alone. Many of us are food addicts. We need to take this into account when we try to alter our eating behavior.

The best way to understand addiction, or addictive behavior, is to think of that behavior as a reflex. When the doctor taps your knee with a reflex hammer, the leg reflexively jumps. The hammer's impact triggers an automatic response that is difficult to control.

Eating addiction involves a similar process.

When we are addicted to food, our behaviors around food, as well as our feelings of hunger, become part of an automatic circuit. A switch gets turned on, like a reflex, and off we go. We think we are hungry and we eat as part of an automatic pathway in our brain, not because our bodies need more energy. But, with effort, we can disrupt that circuitry. We can create new, healthier pathways in the brain that overpower these abnormal ones.

But it takes effort. It takes motivation. And it may take feeling hungry to do it. It may take discipline, resolve, and willpower. It may be difficult.

So remember, when we are trying to change our food behaviors, to eat less than we previously ate, our food-addicted brains will tell us not to change. But it is important and necessary to work through these moments without giving in. That is how we can change how we eat. We can change our behaviors around food and overcome our food addictions.

Most people tell me that there is a period of time, usually 2 to 4 weeks, when they experience a great deal of stress sticking to their new eating goals, but that with time, it becomes easier. There are obvious parallels between this and the experience of alcoholics who try to stop drinking and smokers who try to quit. It is part of the very same process.

Therefore, at least in this respect, it may be necessary to feel some hunger when you are trying to initiate a significant change in the way you eat and lose weight.

Does that mean it will be necessary to go starving for months on end? It does not. That is not advisable because it is not likely to be sustainable. But early in the process you may do well to expect, and maybe even benefit from, some level of hunger. After an initial induction period, the body should adjust, and those feelings should occur less often and with less intensity.

Weight Loss Medications and Supplements

Just as we all hope to find that magic diet that allows us to eat what we want, go hunger free, avoid the gym, and still lose weight, we also hold out hope for the magic of weight loss through pharmaceuticals.

Because I am a physician, you might expect that I would be enthusiastic about this topic. I am not. But I am open to the possibility that an effective and safe weight loss supplement or medication could come along in the future. So far, though, the history of weight loss medication has been disappointing. Most of the medications used for this purpose in the past have come up short on sustained weight loss and long on adverse effects.

The most well-known weight loss medication fiasco occurred in the late 1990s with the drug combination fenfluramine/phentermine, usually called fen-phen, which caused great controversy (and legal issues) when it was found to cause significant heart and lung damage.

The market for weight loss medications cooled down significantly for the next 15 years, but over the last couple of years, a number of prescription weight loss medications have been approved by the Food and Drug Administration (FDA) and reached the market.

I summarize the current state of these new medications as follows: the weight loss effects associated with newer prescription weight loss medications are inconsistent, and for those who do lose weight, the amount of weight is often not very significant. That being said, newer weight loss medications, if they are combined (and only if they are combined) with healthy eating and regular exercise, may help some people achieve more significant weight loss.

As for their safety, it is too early to say.

What Really Works for Weight Loss

It goes without saying that weight control and weight loss are challenging for many, if not most, of us. It is important to be prepared to work hard and to have as many tools available as possible to help ensure your success.

But what really works best when it comes to weight loss?

The best-informed answer comes from the work of the National Weight Control Registry (NWCR). Since 1994, the NWCR has followed a large number of people who have successfully lost weight. First and foremost, "findings from the National Weight Control Registry underscore the fact that it is possible to achieve and maintain significant amounts of weight loss."

Their research reveals the following information about study participants who have lost weight:

- Forty-five percent of participants lost the weight on their own, and the other 55 percent lost weight with the help of some type of program.
- Ninety-eight percent of participants report that they modified their food intake in some way to lose weight.
- Ninety-four percent increased their physical activity, with the most frequently reported form of activity being walking.
- There is variety in how NWCR members keep the weight off. Most report continuing to maintain a low-calorie, low-fat diet and doing high levels of activity.
  - Seventy-eight percent eat breakfast every day.
  - Seventy-five percent weigh themselves at least once a week.
  - Sixty-two percent watch less than 10 hours of TV per week.
  - Ninety percent exercise, on average, about 1 hour per day.

Conclusions

Weight loss is possible, and it is best accomplished through a combination of decreased calorie intake and increased physical activity.

It is more difficult to control our weight or to lose weight with diet alone, or with exercise alone. A combination of the two is best.

Tony Horton, creator of the famed P90X fitness system, says, "You can't outrun a bad diet! Exercise and eating go hand in hand."

Losing weight may not be easy for many of us, but it can be done.

The point is that you should be prepared for a challenge and must be motivated and committed to making real change.

The *Be Healthy! Workbook* will help you with a simple plan to change your eating and increase exercise.

You will track your progress with periodic weigh-ins and mirror checks. You will learn what works for you. If what you are doing is not producing the results you expect, then be prepared to change your approach until you are successful.

Chapter 10

Nutrition 101

One of the most important goals of the *Be Healthy! Workbook* is to help you to improve your eating. More than anything else we can control, our food and eating choices can increase our odds of living a long and healthy life and lower our odds of developing serious illness. Most of the *Be Healthy! Workbook* focuses on how much you eat, but what you eat is just as important.

Unfortunately, many of us struggle to understand and keep up with nutritional science and the most recent recommendations for optimal eating. To make matters worse, there seem to be many controversies and conflicting recommendations when it comes to nutrition.

This brief section will help you sort things out.

Nutrition in a Nutshell: Keeping It Simple
Here's what we know for sure:

1. Vegetables and fruit are good for you.
2. We eat too much.

So here is nutrition in a nutshell. Eat less. Eat more vegetables and fruit. If you read no further, you already have most of the information you need to know!

Further, among dietary approaches that have been studied, the Mediterranean diet appears to offer the most benefits. The Mediterranean diet is rich in fresh vegetables and fruit, whole grains, olive oil, fish and seafood, beans, nuts, legumes, seeds, herbs, and spices.

What else do we know? We know that certain foods are probably not good for us. Sugars, especially high fructose corn syrup, are not good. Partially hydrogenated fats, found in many commercial snack foods, are not good.

So now, here's nutrition in a nutshell:

1. Eat less.
2. Eat more vegetables and fruit.
3. Fill in the rest of your diet emphasizing whole grains, olive oil, fish and seafood, beans, nuts, legumes, seeds, herbs, and spices.
4. Avoid most sweets, sugary beverages, commercial snack foods, and junk foods.

That, my friends, is what we need to know about nutrition. Nutrition seems more complicated than that, doesn't it? But it isn't!

It seems more complicated because there have been, and still are, a number of controversies regarding optimal nutrition.

Nutrition Controversies

Nutrition seems more complicated primarily because of food marketing, a number of well-known controversies over the years, and a healthy dose of legitimate scientific questions that remain.

Food marketing creates complications regarding nutrition because food marketers want you to buy their products. Therefore, they make lots of claims about their food products that may not be true. That's called marketing! And they're good at it. And yes, there have been a number of seemingly confusing controversies over the years regarding particular foods and their health benefits (or negative health effects).

- So first we were told that eggs were bad. Now they're OK.

- Then we were told that butter was bad. It was replaced by margarine. Then it turned out that margarine was bad. Now butter is probably better again.

- Then we were told that we ate too much protein (meat and fat) and that lower-calorie carbs would help us control our weight. Then we heard the opposite, that carbs are the cause of excessive weight gain. This issue remains unsettled.

- We were told that fat was bad, especially saturated fat, the type of fat found in red meats. Now the issue is less clear. There may be good fats (monounsaturated fats, found in vegetable oils, seafood, and nuts) and bad fats (like saturated and partially hydrogenated fats). But a recent large study found no problems associated with the intake of saturated fats!

- Coffee was supposed to be bad for you. Now it appears it may be good for you. Hurray!

- For years, we have been sold on the benefits of supplements and vitamins, and many of us take all manner of vitamins and all sorts of miracle supplements and herbs. None of them have ever been proven to be of benefit, and some may cause harm.

Is there a way to make sense of it all? I think there is.

It's written above already. Our diets should focus on vegetables and fruits. We should consume fewer calories overall. We should emphasize the foods found in the Mediterranean diet. Avoid sugary foods and beverages, and most commercial junk and snack foods.

When it comes to the rest, those foods mentioned above as controversial, such as meat, butter, and eggs, remember, everything in moderation. It's OK to eat them and enjoy them. But they should be eaten in moderation. Eggs, butter, and red meat should not make up a large portion of your daily food intake.

What about carbs? I find that the concept of *nutritional density* is helpful in making decisions regarding carbs and many other food choices.

Nutritional Density

Nutritional density refers to the nutrient quantity that a food contains per calorie (Nutritional Density = Nutrient Content/Calorie). Nutrient-dense foods contain the most nutrients for the fewest calories. In other words, nutrient-dense foods give you the most nutritional value at the expense of the fewest calories.

We want to eat the foods that are the most nutrient rich but contain the fewest calories. Most vegetables, beans, and fresh fruits are good examples of foods that are high in nutritional density.

We want to eat less of foods that have little nutritional value but a large number of calories. These are the "empty calories" so often referred to. A perfect example of a food choice with low nutritional density is soda—or almost any other sweet snack or beverage you can think of. Those foods have no nutritional value for the calories you consume.

Using nutritional density as a guide, we can make decisions about breads and other carbs. White breads and other highly refined carbs have low nutritional density. Much of the nutritional value has been ground out and removed. Therefore, white bread should not make up a large part of your diet. Even breads made from unprocessed whole grains (which have more nutritional value) are still relatively high in calories, so they are not the best choice on the nutritional density scale.

In other words, we should probably eat less white bread (and other "whites," such as white rice or pasta). Whole grains and breads are better, but should not receive nearly the emphasis that vegetables, beans, and fruits should.

I will also make a special note here for people who have diabetes. There is some evidence, and my patients' experience seems to support this claim, that eating highly refined carbs, such as white breads, rice, and pastas (and my patients mention potatoes, as well) makes it more difficult to control blood sugar. Many of my patients have achieved better blood sugar control by avoiding these foods.

Like many nutritional rating scales (the glycemic index would be another popular nutrition rating scale), though, the concept of nutritional density has its controversies and limitations. It is difficult (and controversial) to quantify a food's true nutrient value. Recognizing such limitations, I still like the general concept of nutritional density, which makes it clear why most plant-based foods are better eating choices than sugary, highly processed and refined foods, and junk and snack foods.

Supplements

Shouldn't we all be taking fish oil, Vitamin D, CoQ-10, and every other herb and supplement that is supposed to be the next magic bullet? The answer is probably not.

I have not seen any convincing evidence that any supplement has proven benefit. There *have* been studies that have shown *potential harms* for multivitamins and Vitamin E. The following scenario has been replicated multiple times (see antioxidant vitamins/Vitamins A, C, E, Vitamin D, fish oil):

- First, studies show that a medical condition is associated with a *vitamin deficiency* in the body.
- Based on those studies, we presume that giving the vitamin or supplement in pill form will correct the corresponding medical condition.
- As a result, people begin taking massive amounts of the vitamin/supplement in pill form.
- And finally, clinical studies show that replacing the deficiency with the vitamin/substance in pill form yields no actual health benefits.

The bottom line is that nutrients found in foods have so far not been shown to be of benefit when they are packaged in pill form.

So there is no magic bullet. In other words, there is no vitamin or supplement that we can take that will make or keep us healthy. Making matters worse, many people take supplements because they seem like the path of least resistance to becoming healthy. They feel that they can take a supplement to make up for their dietary indiscretions and lack of exercise. To the best of our knowledge, this is just not accurate. Healthy foods, healthy eating behaviors, and exercise are all necessary aspects of being healthy.

Finally, I will gripe about supplements from the perspective of a practicing mainstream physician. As I mentioned earlier, many people will take any manner of supplements in the mistaken belief that they are "natural" and must be safe and, at the same time, fear prescribed medications like the plague, presuming that they must be unsafe since they are manmade.

First of all, very few supplements are actually "natural." Second, even if they are natural, that doesn't mean the supplement is beneficial or benign. I wish things were so simple.

Conclusion

Our food and eating choices can keep us healthy or make us sick. What foods we eat and how much we eat are both extremely important things to consider, and yet we should try not to obsess about one food that may be evil or one that is touted as a miracle. Nutritional science is just not advanced to the point that such claims are justified. "Everything in moderation" is still a decent guide to making food choices. Also, even though it is of the utmost importance that we make good food and eating choices, food is also something that can and should be enjoyed!

I find a wonderful, exceedingly simple way to think about food choices is to divide my dinner plate into 4 quarters. In the old days, the plate would have been ¾ meat/main course and ¼ vegetable/healthy stuff (if that). There was probably a hunk of tasty bread somewhere, as well.

Today it is the exact opposite: ¾ of the plate should be filled with vegetables/fruit/beans (healthy stuff) and ¼ with a healthy "main dish" (see Image 14). I try to eat smaller portions (on a smaller plate), and there is usually no bread (and no seconds).

It's simple!

Oh, and if a new study comes out and all of this information changes, I apologize. It is a fast-moving society that we live in, and when it comes to science, health, and especially nutrition, the reality is that change happens!

In the space below, write down any issues you have with eating and nutrition, and ways you may improve how you eat.

_____

_____

_____

_____

_____

_____

_____

_____

Chapter 11

Assignment: Controlling Eating Behavior

This is a mandatory section/assignment.

Many, if not most, of us have trouble controlling ourselves when we get around food. We especially have trouble controlling ourselves around the foods we love (but are not supposed to love). Many people tell me that they eat too quickly, and before they know it, have eaten too much. But to optimize our health, it is important that we gain control over our eating behaviors. This section is intended to help you get control of your eating. The following is a menu of techniques that you can use to help gain control over your eating habits and behavior. You may try any or all of them. Find what works for you.

You may notice that many of the techniques are similar to those used to help smokers stop smoking and alcoholics stop drinking. That is because many of our eating behaviors are similar to other types of addictive behavior. In other words, many of us are food addicts. One of the reasons that so many people fail in their attempts to improve their eating is that we fail to understand this very important fact. So:

- Remove all trigger/problem foods and beverages from your home and your usual surroundings (like work, if possible). Many of us, if we have easy access to snack and junk foods, sweets, and sugary juices and sodas, will consume them. Having easy access serves as an uncontrollable eating/drinking trigger. Avoidance is a good way to begin to gain control. Avoid the temptation by ridding your home and usual surroundings of temptation. Don't buy them and don't have them around.

- ○ Surround yourself with healthy eating options. As a corollary to removing trigger/problem foods, you should make it as easy as possible to eat good foods. Surround yourself with healthy foods, snacks, and options. For example, I always take berries and bananas to work.

- Relax and get control prior to eating anything. Too many times, when we are stressed and/or hungry, we dive into a snack or meal, and before we know it, have consumed too much food! This may be the easiest and most common thing we can do to comfort ourselves (and it works, right?). We should never begin to eat without first taking a moment to calm ourselves. Try this technique (or come up with your own).

  - ○ For 60 seconds prior to eating anything, breathe deeply, try to relax your mind and body, and even make a quick plan to eat slowly and a moderate amount of food.

- Eat slowly and take a break between each mouthful or bite of food. Just as it is easy to dive too quickly into a meal, and then to overeat, it is also common for many of us, once we get started, to shovel the food into our mouths in a frenzy of over-consumption. We must learn to eat slowly. Try this technique.

  - ○ Put down your fork or spoon after each mouthful of food. Take a breath after you have swallowed a mouthful of food. Slow down. Ask yourself if you have had enough prior to the next bite. Try to stop for a few moments and get a sense of whether you are really still hungry.

- Don't finish what is on your plate. I know that this seems counter to what we have been taught about waste. But learning to finish everything on your plate (my mother told me this, too) is one of the reasons that many of us eat too much. I am not suggesting that you waste a significant amount of food (that would be wrong). First of all, I hope that you are only placing reasonable portions on your plate.

But then, as an exercise in control, try leaving a little bit of food on the plate.

- Have a plan for every meal. Some people may find it helpful to plan, and even write out, a schedule or plan for their daily or weekly meals. In addition, making a mental game plan prior to each meal, detailing what foods and how much you should eat, may be helpful.

- Have a plan for surprises, parties, or unexpected situations or temptations. We all encounter unexpected situations, and many of them can involve food or hunger. It is very easy to lose control in such moments. Having a specific, detailed plan, even a written one, in place that anticipates such moments will go a long way to helping you successfully handle yourself.

- Fill up on the good stuff first. Part of your eating and food control plan may include beginning each meal with healthy, filling vegetables and salad. Satisfy your hunger by slowly eating the most healthful foods available—your vegetables, salads, and fruits. Eat the "entrée" (hopefully a healthy one) only after your urge to eat has mostly been satisfied.

- Avoid grazing. One of today's more popular approaches to eating is to eat small amounts of food throughout the day rather than three large meals. This may be suitable for some people, but it is also an easy way to eat a great deal of food. Especially for those of us who have trouble controlling ourselves around food, grazing (especially without a detailed plan) may not be a good idea.

- Drink water or a little coffee first. Many people have told me that they successfully suppressed their appetite by filling up a large jug of water and drinking good amounts through the day. My personal experience is that a little bit of coffee helps satisfy some of my cravings. On the other hand, I have read that having coffee may result in cravings later on when the caffeine jolt wears off. You should experiment with what works for you.

- Exercise first or throughout the day. There is some research showing that aerobic exercise can curb appetite for a period of time. I have found that exercising in the evening, prior to dinner, has led to a tremendous reduction in my dinner and after-dinner appetite (it has been like a miracle for me). Also, you may try short bursts of exercise, such as a high-intensity interval training (HIIT) workout (see Chapter 19, "Physical Activity," for more about HIIT workouts) throughout the day.

- Brief food fasts. Smokers can stop smoking and drinkers can give up alcohol. We can't give up food, and I don't suggest going on crash diets, where you fast for prolonged periods. On the other hand, avoiding food for brief periods may have certain benefits in helping to reduce food cravings and unhealthy behaviors.

Addiction is wired into the brain. When smokers avoid tobacco, they can partially disconnect those wires. When we fast for brief periods, we may be able to do the same thing to the wiring that affects our eating habits.

I have developed a technique (I call it the "Sabbath Diet") where I fast for one day of the week until sunset. I do this on Saturday or Sunday, hence the "Sabbath Diet." I choose these days because it would not be good to be too hungry while I work, and it is easier for me to be in control on a more relaxed day (the day of rest).

Fasting for one day achieves the following for me: I practice self-control, which has helped me gain more control over my usual eating patterns. And I cut a certain percentage of my weekly calories, which helps me lose and control my weight.

It is extremely important to end the fast (my evening meal) in a very controlled way, with a small meal, eaten slowly, and little (if any) snacking afterwards. This technique has helped me to strengthen my ability to control cravings later in the week.

You may want to try this as well, with the following disclaimer: you should not try this if you suffer from significant hypoglycemia (low sugar events) or take medications that make even a short fast potentially dangerous, like certain medications used to treat diabetes. Also, if you have an eating disorder, such as anorexia, this is not a good idea for you. If there is any question about whether this is a safe technique for you, please consult your physician before attempting it.

- The "12-hour window." Another technique some people use is to allow eating only during certain hours of the day (*New York Times*, 2015). Having such a rule may help reduce snacking and overall calorie intake. Research shows that eating for only 12 hours of the day may encourage weight loss.

    I tried the 8-hour diet (allowed to eat only 8 hours of the day), but I was just too ravenous at work (people noticed, believe me). Twelve hours may be more achievable, effective, and reasonable for many people.

- Enlist a food control buddy. Sometimes it helps to enlist the help of others. Maybe you have a workmate who is also trying to get control of their eating. You can monitor one another and help hold one another accountable to your eating goals. Spouses and other family members are another obvious choice (though I am convinced that my wife attempts to fatten me up so that she looks better than me!).

    My running buddy (Russell) and I use what we refer to as "public shaming." When we need to lose a little weight, we e-mail each other our weights each morning. We find this technique very effective. It is not for everyone, but it may be for you.

- Find the foods that satisfy you. Appetite control is challenging and poorly understood. There remains much to learn. You should find the healthy foods that effectively control your appetite. What works for you may not be the same as what works for others.

    As I've said, for me, it's berries and bananas. I often eat berries on the way home in the evening, which means that I don't walk in the door too hungry. These foods also give me great energy for my evening workout. Some people like apples for this purpose. They take a long time to eat. Carrots are the same way.

More than any other technique mentioned in this section, this one may take personal experimentation. You need to find what works for you, but remember that it should be a healthy choice!

• Get enough sleep. Research shows that people who don't get enough sleep tend to gain weight.

Notes

In the space below, use the techniques detailed above (or you may have your own) to plan how you will attempt to control your eating behaviors. Be as specific as possible, and try to plan for as many situations you may encounter as possible.

Chapter 12

Assignment: Portion Control

A long with "Controlling Your Eating Behaviors," this is a mandatory section.

One of the obvious problems is that we pile too much food on our plates. In this section, we discuss tricks that can help you reduce portion sizes.

What Is a Serving?

First of all, many of us may take too much food because we overestimate the size of a serving. I don't like to get too technical about this, but I do think it is useful to know, at least in general terms, simple ways to estimate a serving of food.

The National Institutes of Health have a nice "Serving Size Card" that includes some simple rules of thumb for estimating the size of a portion. They list the following images to describe a serving of various foods:

- One serving of salad greens = 1 cup = the size of a baseball.
- One serving of fruit = ½ cup = half the size of a baseball.
- One serving of cereal flakes = 1 cup = the size of a fist.
- One serving of cooked rice or pasta = ½ cup = half the size of a baseball.
- One serving of meat, fish, or poultry = 3 ounces = a deck of cards.

- One serving of peanut butter = 2 tablespoons = the size of a ping pong ball.
- One serving of cheese = 1½ ounces = 4 stacked dice or 2 slices.

I think the point is that these "servings" are smaller than what most of us think of as a serving, or portion.

The simplest message I can think of, and the best way to reduce your portion size, is to take or eat portions that are smaller than the ones you currently eat. If the idea is to reduce your weight by reducing the amount of food that you currently consume, you need to eat portions that are smaller than the ones you currently eat. That's a pretty simple way to look at it.

Some people also suggest that measuring foods out (using an actual measuring cup) can be of help, as well. Especially when you are just setting out on your portion control journey, this can be useful.

Use Smaller Plates, Bowls, and Glasses

I really love this idea. Use smaller plates, bowls, and glasses. What appeals to me is how simple an approach this is. There is no measuring and no estimating portion size. The small plate simply limits the amount you can eat (be careful not to pile your food skyward in an attempt to overcome the small plate size).

And filling up a small plate, as opposed to partially filling a large plate, may create the illusion that we are eating more than we think.

A really nice approach is to use portion control plates, which are divided into appropriately sized sections for the different food types.

I will sometimes eat dinner on a saucer-size plate. If I go to a party or special event, I allow myself to fill one saucer-size plate with food. I try to eat very slowly. This works great for me and has enabled me to substantially reduce the amount of food I eat.

The "No Seconds" Rule

This is a pretty obvious approach, but I like simple rules to help us make good eating decisions.

In addition to eating smaller portions, once you are done, you are done. It's a shame when you have gone through the trouble of preparing a healthy meal, eat a healthy amount, but then add a second (or third) portion, undoing your efforts. In other words, two small portions equal a large portion. No second helpings!

Avoid Family-Style Dining and All-You-Can-Eat Restaurants

Don't transfer the food from the stove to a serving bowl to the table. Having a bowl (or bowls) of essentially unlimited amounts of food right in front of you on the table ("family style") is too tempting. Keep the food on the stove. Portion the food on your (small) plate directly from the pot on the stove and then take it to the table (out of easy reach). It might help.

Also, just avoid all-you-can-eat situations. Don't go to all-you-can-eat restaurants.

Be very careful at potlucks!

If you do end up in one of these situations, go in with a specific plan detailing how much you can eat—and use small plates and bowls!

Eating at Restaurants

Restaurants are a challenge. They make very tasty food, and they tend to serve huge amounts of it.

The best idea I have heard is to share an order between two people. That's really enough food. Another approach that I like is to divide your plate in two and only eat half. You can have the other half boxed or just leave it there. Boxing the rest of the food increases the chances that you will just go home and eat the rest, which will defeat the purpose. I have done that too many times!

I remember the first time I only ate half of my serving at a great restaurant. I felt like I had lost my best buddy (I'm not kidding!).

Andy Warhol on Weight Loss: Choose Foods You Don't Like

"When I order in a restaurant, I order everything that I don't want, so I have a lot to play around with while everyone else eats. Then, no matter how chic the restaurant is, I insist that the waiter wrap the entire plate up like a to-go order, and after we leave the restaurant I find a little corner outside in the street to leave the plate in, because there are so many people in New York who live in the streets, with everything they own in shopping bags. . . . So I lose weight and stay trim, and I think that maybe one of those people will find a Grenouille dinner on the window ledge."

So that's the Andy Warhol New York City Diet.

Final Note

At first, eating smaller portions may be challenging. I miss my larger portions. But smaller portions are not just something that we do while we are reducing weight. It is a key aspect of a healthy lifestyle.

You need to commit to smaller portions, not just in the short term but for life!

Notes

In the space below, plan how you will decrease your portion sizes.

Chapter 13

Assignment: Cutting Snacks, Sweets, and Junk Foods

This assignment is easy for me to write about, but it may be hard for you to read and even harder to accomplish.

If we want to control our weight and maintain our health, we need to get rid of junk and snack foods. For many of us, this may be the most important change we can make, as far as our eating and health are concerned. Many people tell me that they eat chocolates and other sweets, candy, ice cream, chips, cookies, donuts, cakes and pies, and the like, on a daily basis, if not multiple times per day. However, most, if not all, common snack foods are bad in at least two ways:

- They add extra, unnecessary calories. A lot of them.
- They contain sugars, refined carbs, and chemicals that may be harmful.

The number one trending concept in nutritional science right now is that refined (or white) carbohydrates and sugars (high-fructose corn syrup may be the worst) rather than fats may be the most harmful food components in our diets. These are the biggest components in many of the snacks and junk foods that we eat.

But for those who consume large amounts of snacks, sweets, and junk foods, avoiding them is one of the easiest and most effective ways to lose weight and improve nutrition and overall health.

For many, though, eliminating their cherished donuts, chips, and ice cream from their diets may be difficult because these foods, more than any others, are the focus of food addictions. Also, these foods taste great.

Initially, complete avoidance may be the key to success. For many people, if there is easy access to snacks, chips, junk foods, and sweets, the temptation will be too great. Therefore, the first step needs to be banishing all junk foods and snacks from your home. You may want to do the same thing in your workplace as well. Perhaps your workmates will support you.

One of the offices where I worked seemed to have parties offering sweets and junk foods every day. It was so easy, mid-morning or mid-afternoon, to grab a cookie or two, or a piece of cake. Soon I noticed I was gaining weight. The staff bristled when I suggested we rid the office of all the junk.

Eventually, I used a little mind trick to keep me from going for the junk. I told myself that junk foods, candies, and snack foods weren't food at all. "Food," as I had redefined it, was only the kinds of food that could help me stay and be healthy.

In my new frame of mind, snacks, sweets, and junk foods were viewed as poison. I also used the idea of junk foods as a gun with very slow bullets, imagining that each time I ate junk I was pulling the trigger. Another helpful image I used was of snack and junk foods as stuffing. All these foods would do was stuff me, or make me bigger, like a Thanksgiving turkey.

These images, and my changed mind-set concerning snack and junk foods, really helped me stop putting them in my mouth! I went long periods without touching any junk foods, which was a big change and a big victory for me.

Another way that you may mentally reframe the snack and junk foods that you regularly consume is to view them as rare "treats." A treat is something that you get in rare instances, like special occasions, or as a reward for some important milestone or accomplishment. Under such circumstances, a "treat" might be something that you would consume less than once per week (or once per month).

That is the nature of this very important, life-changing, if not life-saving, assignment.

It's simple. Stop most, if not all, sweets, junk foods snacks, cookies, candies, chips, crackers, cakes, donuts, pies, ice cream, and so on.

It's really important!

Notes/Ideas/Comments/Plans

In the space below, plan how you will cut down on or eliminate specific snacks/sweets/junk foods.

Chapter 14

Assignment: Stopping Night Eating

E ating after the dinner meal, through the evening, and even through the night is extremely common. After sweets and junk food, after-dinner and night eating is the most common eating problem that my patients tell me about.

It is a substantial problem for many people, adding hundreds (if not thousands) of unnecessary calories per night. For many, it is a difficult behavior to control.

Many people tell me that soon after they finish the dinner meal, they develop an almost uncontrollable hunger that results in excessive snacking. For them, after-dinner eating and snacking are both the cause of their weight issues and also the path to a relatively simple solution. Stop eating after dinner!

Of course, it is simple for me to write that you should stop eating after dinner. It may be far more difficult for you to actually stop.

Did you ever wonder why you felt so hungry shortly after eating what for many of us is the biggest meal of the day? Do you know in your head that you shouldn't be hungry, but still feel hungry and end up eating anyway? Do you have trouble stopping yourself? Do you end up eating far more than you intended? The fact is that our eating behaviors are complicated. And many of us are food addicts.

You should be ready, therefore, when you decide to cut back or stop your after-dinner eating, to experience resistance. Your body will try to convince you that you are making some type of mistake. You will feel hungry. You may feel anxious. You may feel like you are missing a friend.

That is the body's way of fighting any significant change in eating behavior. You should put yourself in the best possible situation to encourage successful change.

Avoid eating triggers. First and foremost, get rid of temptation by getting your typical after-dinner snacks out of the house.

Get busy. Boredom is the number one reason people tell me they start eating after dinner.

Don't sit in front of the TV right after dinner. The combination of a couch or comfortable chair and a TV after dinner creates a powerful, seemingly subliminal pull toward the refrigerator or snack drawer.

I find that exercising in the evening helps control my hunger.

I also really like using the "12-hour window rule," mentioned in the "Controlling Eating Behavior" chapter. This rule allows food consumption for only 12 hours of the day, like 7:00 a.m. to 7:00 p.m. At 7:00 p.m., no matter what, no more food. I have found this to be a simple and effective way to gain control over after-dinner eating.

Again, be ready for a battle. But also know that after a short time, an induction period that usually lasts 2 to 4 weeks, it should become easier.

For more tips on controlling eating behaviors, see Chapter 11, "Controlling Eating Behavior."

As an assignment, create a plan for cutting back on or stopping your after-dinner food consumption.

_____

_____

_____

_____

_____

_____

_____

Chapter 15

Assignment: Cutting Beverage Sugar and Calories

Many people do not realize that what they drink can affect their health in just the same way as the solid foods they eat. They get a tremendous amount of sugar and calories from beverages like soda, juice, milk, alcohol, sweetened tea, and energy drinks. Many patients reveal to me that they drink huge numbers of both alcoholic and non-alcoholic beverages, adding hundreds, if not thousands, of calories per day! Some people are overweight solely because of what they drink.

It's a problem.

There's an easy solution, of course. Stop drinking beverages with sugar or calories. Water has neither sugar nor calories. Drink water only.

If the beverages you overconsume contain caffeine, cut back gradually. Going cold turkey can create a nasty headache and other symptoms of caffeine withdrawal.

As an assignment, create a plan to decrease or to stop entirely drinking beverages with sugar or calories.

Chapter 16

Assignment: Fast Food and Restaurant Eating

Many people eat out for a large portion of their meals, and many of those meals are at fast food restaurants.

There are many issues with fast food. By definition, it is fast. It is often ordered when we are in a hurry and eaten in a hurry. It is, therefore, easy to eat a lot of food in a short amount of time. Also, fast food is often high in calorie counts (super-sized) and low on nutrition scores.

As for non–fast food restaurants, the biggest issue is portion size. Many restaurants pile a lot of food on oversized plates. Compounding the issue, there are often unlimited drinks, appetizers, and desserts. If you are someone who eats out a lot, there are three options:

1. Eat out less often.
2. Choose healthier options when you eat out.
3. Eat less when you eat out.

Eating out less often may be the best option. Many of us just find it too challenging to avoid overeating and ordering the "bad— but very tasty—stuff" when we eat out.

If, however, you are someone who eats out because of a challenging schedule, it may be necessary to use some planning and creativity in order to get more meals at home (or from home).

But eating out is a great American tradition and can also be the source of fine food, which is one of life's great pleasures.

If you do eat out, try to make healthier choices. Most restaurants, even fast-food restaurants and convenience stores, now carry healthier food items. Also, if you eat out, plan to eat less. For instance, one simple strategy is to eat only half of what is served on the plate. Or, share one meal between two people. See Chapter 11, "Controlling Eating Behavior" for more ideas.

As an assignment, write a plan for dealing with restaurant and fast food eating.

Chapter 17

Assignment: Reducing White Breads, Pastas, and Refined Carbs

Whether you believe that carbs are "good" or carbs are "bad," I would argue that they should not make up a large percentage of our dietary food intake. Highly refined carbohydrates—the white breads, rice, and pastas—score low on ratings of nutritional density. They have little nutritional value per calorie.

In addition, refined carbohydrates may encourage weight gain and increase glucose and insulin levels, especially in people who are more susceptible to this (those with diabetes and the metabolic syndrome).

I think of breads, rice, and pastas as "stuffing." They do relatively little for us nutritionally, but they add on the pounds. But they are tasty, aren't they? Who doesn't love a plate of spaghetti, accompanied by good Italian or French bread?

But, alas, if we are concerned about our weight and our overall health, only the best foods (that is, those with the highest nutritional density like vegetables and fruit) earn their way into our bodies. There just isn't a lot of room in a healthy diet for a lot of extras.

So if you are someone who tends to eat a lot of bread and pasta, and especially if you have trouble controlling your weight or you are a diabetic struggling with blood sugar control, you should reduce that amount in your diet.

In our household (my wife, daughter, and I were strict vegetarians for years), where we used to eat pasta and rice multiple times per week and where bread used to accompany many meals, those amounts have declined drastically. And while sandwiches were once a staple of our lunchtime eating, I now eat many of the foods that were previously packed between two slices of bread, like turkey or chicken, sliced up into a much more nutritionally dense (and still very tasty) salad.

If you are someone who eats a lot of refined carbohydrates in the form of bread, rice, and pasta, use the space below to plan how you will reduce or eliminate some or most of those foods from your diet.

Chapter 18

Assignment: Optimal Nutrition

Much of the *Be Healthy! Workbook* is devoted to eliminating certain types of foods, excessive calories, and harmful eating behaviors. But optimal nutrition is as much about what we do eat as what we don't eat. In fact, it may be more important to eat healthier foods than avoid harmful ones.

So at the same time that we are eliminating harmful aspects of our diets and overeating, we need to increase the percentage of the best foods, vegetables, fruits, and beans that comprise our diets. There are some easy approaches to this goal.

I try to have some fruit with every breakfast, and fruit is my primary form of mid-morning, mid-afternoon, and after-work snacks. I bring two bananas, and usually assorted other fruits, like apples, grapes, or pineapple, to work with me.

I also eat a super nutritious salad at lunch.

Then, at dinner, I apply the ¾ of the plate vegetables and salad and ¼ of the plate healthy entrée plate rule.

That's a lot of vegetables and fruit!

Remember, in the "Nutrition 101" section, we advised you to:

1. Eat less.
2. Eat more vegetables and fruit.
3. Fill in the rest of your diet emphasizing whole grains, olive oil, fish and seafood, beans, nuts, legumes, seeds, herbs and spices.

4. Avoid most sweets, sugary beverages, commercial snack foods, and junk foods.

Through a number of assignments, the *Be Healthy! Workbook* helped you remove the foods you shouldn't eat.

The next step is to analyze what you *are* eating.

In the space below, plan how you will improve the nutritional content of your diet (in other words, how you will get lots of vegetables, salads, fruit, legumes, unrefined cereals, and fish into your diet).

Chapter 19

Assignment: Physical Activity

R emember two important points:

1. The great majority of people who lose weight and keep it off exercise a lot.
2. Being sedentary can kill you!

The goal is to take you from wherever you are currently on the physical activity and exercise continuum and to increase until you are doing as much as you can on as many days per week, at the highest intensity level possible (all within reason, of course).

This chapter contains information and answers to questions that will help you get to that goal.

How Much Exercise Is Enough?

The Centers for Disease Control and Prevention (CDC) recommends:

- At least 150 minutes per week (a little over 20 minutes per day) of moderate-intensity aerobic activity (or 75 minutes per week of vigorous intensity aerobic activity) *and*
- Muscle-strengthening activities on at least 2 days per week.

That seems like a reasonable place to start.

Also consider that the more you do, the more you may benefit. A recent study showed that compared with someone who does not exercise, someone over the age of 40 who walks briskly for 75 minutes per week (just over 10 minutes per day) can add 1.8 years to their life expectancy. But more exercise adds more benefit. Walking briskly for at least 450 minutes per week (just over an hour per day) was associated with a gain of 4.5 years.

So how much exercise is enough? The answer depends on a number of factors. For our purposes, let's assume that you are attempting to lose weight *and* that you would like to add as many healthy, active years to your life as possible. Under those circumstances, a reasonable initial goal would be to exercise at least 30 minutes per day—and ultimately 30 to 60 minutes per day—at a moderate to vigorous intensity level. You should also aim to include muscle strengthening at least 2 days per week.

However, if you find that the above goal of 30 minutes per day of at least moderate-intensity exercise, when combined with your eating goals, does not result in adequate weight loss, you may need to increase either the amount of exercise you do or the intensity level.

Also, if you have not been exercising regularly or if you have any health conditions, the general advice is start low and go slow with your changes. This will help you avoid injury.

Of course, you should consult your physician prior to beginning any physical activity or exercise program, especially if you have any serious health conditions like high blood pressure, diabetes, or heart disease or you are over the age of 40, have a family history of heart problems, or have not been exercising regularly. Over time, you will get a sense of what your body is capable of and how hard you can push yourself. But at first, as I already said, start low and go slow.

Does Exercise Intensity Matter?

Intensity does matter. One minute of vigorous-intensity exercise is worth 2 minutes of moderate-intensity exercise. Just from a time perspective, the level of exercise intensity matters because you may be able to achieve benefits in less time. For busy individuals, that may make a great difference.

Exercising at a higher intensity level may have other benefits. More intense exercise over a short period may create more weight loss than exercising for a longer duration at a low-intensity rate.

Vigorous physical activity reduces the risk of cardiovascular disease and sudden death more than low-intensity exercise.

That being said, it is not necessary to push yourself past what you are capable of or what you are comfortable with. *Any exercise is better than none.* The intent here is to get you to exercise as much as you can, at the highest level of intensity at which you are comfortable. But remember, increasing your exercise intensity can improve your health and fitness level, and it may save you time. Over time, with regular physical activity, you may be able to add more intense exercise or a mix of moderate and intense physical activity.

Does All the Exercise Have to Occur at the Same Time?

No. Exercise can be broken up into short bursts, and there may even be certain benefits to short bursts of physical activity throughout the day. You can get the same benefits from 10 minutes of exercise 3 or 4 times per day as you can from 30 to 40 minutes of continuous exercise.

In addition, short bursts of intense exercise throughout the day may be even better for weight loss than one long round of moderate-intensity exercise.

What Types of Exercise Activities Are Best?

All types of exercise are good, as long as you do them and the exercise includes at least a moderate level of intensity and focuses on both cardiovascular health and muscle strengthening.

The Centers for Disease Control and Prevention (CDC) defines moderate-intensity aerobic activity as exerting yourself hard enough to raise your heart rate and break a sweat. With moderate-intensity exercise, you can talk but not sing the words to your favorite song. Some examples of activities that require moderate effort are:

- Walking fast
- Doing water aerobics
- Riding a bike on level ground or with few hills
- Playing doubles tennis
- Pushing a lawn mower

The CDC describes vigorous-intensity aerobic activity as exercise that makes you breathe hard and fast and increases your heart rate quite a bit. With vigorous intensity, you won't be able to say more than a few words without pausing for a breath. Some examples of activities that require vigorous effort are:

- Jogging or running
- Swimming laps
- Riding a bike fast or on hills
- Playing singles tennis
- Playing basketball

The most important point to make is that you should be doing *both* aerobic and muscle-strengthening activities to reach optimal health. Traditionally, for many people, to exercise (especially if you were attempting to lose weight) means only to do aerobic activity.

First of all, muscle-strengthening activities can provide an excellent aerobic workout.

Second, muscle-strengthening activities are necessary. Strong muscles protect joints from injury, and they can compensate for damaged joints. The best treatments for arthritis of the hips and knees are weight loss and muscle strengthening.

Most important, strong muscles are the best protection against aging. In fact, I refer to muscle-strengthening exercise as the fountain of youth. I mentioned before that the strongest indication to me that one of my patients is "aging" is that they tell me they can no longer do the things they once liked to do. They can no longer go shopping, take steps, go on trips, or do outdoor chores or other activities. That is most often because of muscle weakness.

Because of that, your exercise activities should include *both* aerobic and muscle-strengthening activities.

Today, you have so many great options, too. Take it from someone who used to think of exercise as running on most days and lifting weights on a few others. There are many more options than that!

In addition to traditional continuous walking, running, and bicycling workouts, there is interval training, where you combine a short period of very high-intensity training with a slower recovery period. There are classes that include multiple forms of yoga, Pilates, dance styles of all kinds, boot camps, big ball, Zumba, cycling, Cross-Fit, kickboxing, martial arts, undulation ropes, and more. There are gyms and workout facilities of all types.

There are all manner of cardiovascular machines, including:

- Treadmills
- Stationary bikes: traditional and recumbent
- Stair stepper machines
- Elliptical trainers
- Stepmills
- Versa climbers
- Tread climbers
- Incline trainers
- Rowing machines
- Hand ergometer

For strength training, there are traditional free weights and weight machines, resistance bands, dumbbell exercises, and body weight exercises (using no weights).

There are core workouts, cross-training workouts, CrossFit, high-intensity interval training (HIIT) workouts, and more.

HIIT workouts are hot right now. They offer the benefit of shorter-duration workouts that can be done almost any time or any place, which makes them great options for people who don't have a lot of time, or who want to add extra exercise to their day. They offset the harmful effects of long sedentary periods. A quick Internet search for HIIT workouts will yield a bounty of great workouts. For a couple of examples, see Image 15.

For those who like to work out at home, there are thousands of exercise videos and DVDs. I tell patients to simply google any type of workout they may be interested in, based on their personal interest, age, and limiting factors like injuries, and something will come up. There are single workouts and entire fitness systems.

Years ago, the Jane Fonda tapes brought fitness options to the home (I admit to doing the Challenge workout many years back, which was very embarrassing at the time; it was a fantastic workout that I could never finish).

I have trained for years doing the P90X workouts (I am a devotee), and I love the Insanity and T25 workouts; both are well-known video-based workout systems developed by fitness instructor Shawn T. and marketed by Beachbody.com. These workouts have transformed my fitness. I also have lots of patients who love the Jillian Michaels workouts.

The point is, there are options for everyone, every age, every interest, every desired level of intensity, indoor or outdoor, gym or home.

In other words, there are no excuses not to exercise every day. I stress to patients that it is most important to have a plan (see below) that enables you to exercise every day, under any circumstances. Focus on the types of exercise that you enjoy!

Exercising with Injuries and Pain

One of the more common reasons that people stop or avoid exercise is pain or injury. The most common scenario my patients describe is that they abandon a walking regimen because of problems related to the knee, hip, or ankle and foot.

A vicious cycle then often develops where, because they are injured or having pain, they aren't exercising. Then, they gain weight, which makes the pain worse, making it even harder to exercise. While it may be more challenging to get and stay fit if you have knee/hip/ankle pain, it is still quite possible. Many people who have pain with walking or jogging can still get a great cardiovascular workout with:

- Swimming
- Elliptical machines (very little stress on the joints)
- Stationary bikes
- Water aerobics
- Pilates
- Tai chi

In addition, most people who have a lower body injury can still perform a great many strength-training exercises, like lifting weights or core exercise routines. And, as stated previously, an intense strength training (especially with low weights and high reps) or core workout can provide an excellent cardiovascular workout as well.

Specific exercises may even be key to helping or fixing the underlying problem causing the pain. The best treatment for osteoarthritis pain is strengthening the muscles around the painful joint and losing weight to decrease the burden on the painful area.

With the types of fitness facilities and home equipment available today, it should be possible to find ways to exercise despite an injury or joint pain. If you are having difficulty finding options, consult a trainer at the gym, a physical therapist, or just google your specific issue. Often, if a patient of mine mentions an injury that is keeping them from exercise, I can just google the issue and have numerous web pages and videos come up, giving them all manner of options.

The only word of caution is that you should not perform an exercise if it is causing significant pain. In other words, if it hurts, don't do it.

Plan to Exercise Under All Conditions

The key is to have a plan. Having a written plan is even better (if it helps you to be more accountable).

To be fit, you must be prepared to exercise almost every day. You need to have options available for indoors and outdoors, bad weather of all types, at home or at some fitness facility available to you.

The most common excuse I hear is that people stop being physically active because it is too cold. I tell them they need to have a plan to stay active 365 days per year.

The second most common problem I hear preventing exercise is that someone is just too busy with work, family, or school. As my grade school industrial arts teacher, Mr. Jacobs, used to say, "I feel for you, but I ain't reachin." In other words, I understand the issue, but I can't accept that as an excuse. Exercise and physical activity are necessary and need to be made a priority.

With some thought and a plan, you can find available times and days of the week when you can exercise. As discussed previously, HIIT workouts enable you to squeeze a great deal of fitness into a short amount of time. Three 10-minute HIIT workouts in a day are equal to 30 minutes of intense exercise!

Conclusion/Assignment

Remember, your ultimate goal is to exercise at least 30 to 60 minutes per day at a moderate to vigorous level of intensity (or the highest level of intensity you are capable of) and to include strength training on at least two days per week.

You need to create a plan to get from where you are currently, in terms of exercise duration and level of intensity, to your goal.

The objective of the *Be Healthy! Workbook* is to take you from wherever you may be today on the exercise/physical activity/fitness spectrum and get you to an optimal level. Regular exercise is an essential (unavoidable) part of being healthy.

If you don't exercise, you need to begin exercising. If you exercise a little, you need to increase that amount. You can increase the duration or frequency of your exercise sessions, or increase the intensity, or add a different type of exercise.

You should be trying to achieve both cardiovascular fitness and muscle strengthening. Many forms of fitness will give you both at the same time.

In the space below, write out a plan to optimize your exercise and physical activity regimen. Focus on increasing your exercise duration, frequency, and/or intensity. Plan for all types of weather and any other barriers you may encounter. Design HIIT workouts you may use to increase your exercise intensity or squeeze in extra fitness throughout the day or when your schedule gets too busy.

Appendix

Supplemental Exercise Plans

Below are sample exercise plans. Feel free to use them in any way you might find helpful.

Sample Plan 1: Appropriate for someone who has not been exercising at all and is beginning the program at a relatively low level of fitness.

Time	Physical Activity Goals
Month 1	Begin walking 30 minutes per day at a comfortable pace. If the weather is bad, substitute home treadmill or stationary bike for any of the walks in this plan.
Month 2	Walk 30 minutes per day at a moderate pace.
Month 3	Walk 30 minutes per day at a moderate pace for 5 days of the week. Begin strength-training workouts at the gym on Monday and Wednesday evenings.
Month 4	Walk 30 minutes per day at a brisk pace for 5 days of the week. Monday and Wednesday evening gym workouts: begin with 9-minute HIIT (treadmill, elliptical, or stationary bike), go 60 seconds hard, rest 60 seconds (repeat 4 more times), followed by full circuit strength workout.

| Month 5 | Walk 30 minutes per day at a brisk pace for 5 days of the week; finish walk with 9-minute walking HIIT workout (walk as fast as possible for 60 seconds; walk slowly for 60 seconds; repeat 4 more times). Monday and Wednesday evening gym workouts: begin with 9-minute HIIT (treadmill, elliptical, or stationary bike), go 60 seconds as hard as possible, rest 60 seconds, followed by full circuit strength workout. |
| Month 6 | Walk 40 minutes per day at a brisk pace for 5 days of the week; finish walk with 9-minute walking HIIT workout (walk as fast as possible for 60 seconds; walk slowly for 60 seconds; repeat 4 more times). Monday and Wednesday evening gym workouts: begin with 9-minute HIIT (treadmill, elliptical, or stationary bike), go 60 seconds as hard as possible, rest 60 seconds, followed by full circuit strength workout. |

Sample Plan 2: Appropriate for someone who has been walking and working out sporadically and is moderately fit, but wants to exercise more regularly and to increase their level of fitness.

Time	Physical Activity Goals
Month 1	Walk 30 minutes per day at a brisk pace (if the weather is bad, substitute home treadmill or other cardio machine for any of the walks in this plan).
Month 2	Begin with 5-minute HIIT/burpee workout (do as many burpees as you can for 30 seconds, and then rest 30 seconds; repeat 4 more times). Walk 30 minutes per day at a brisk pace.
Month 3	Begin with 5-minute HIIT/burpee workout (do as many burpees as you can for 30 seconds, and then rest 30 seconds; repeat 4 more times). Walk 40 minutes per day at a brisk pace. Repeat 5-minute HIIT/burpee workout.

Month 4	Two days per week: intense fitness class or DVD workout. Every other day of the week: begin with 5-minute HIIT/burpee workout (do as many burpees as you can for 30 seconds, and then rest 30 seconds; repeat 4 more times). Walk 40 minutes per day at a brisk pace. Repeat 5-minute HIIT/burpee workout.
Month 5	Three days per week: intense fitness class or home DVD workout. Every other day of the week: begin with 5-minute HIIT/burpee workout (do as many burpees as you can for 30 seconds, and then rest 30 seconds; repeat 4 more times). Walk 40 minutes per day at a brisk pace. Repeat 5-minute HIIT/burpee workout.
Month 6	Three days per week: intense fitness class or home DVD workout. Every other day of the week: begin with 5-minute HIIT/burpee workout (do as many burpees as you can for 30 seconds, and then rest 30 seconds; repeat 4 more times). Walk 50 minutes per day at a brisk pace. Repeat 5-minute HIIT/burpee workout.

Sample Plan 3: Appropriate for someone who has been working out and is moderately fit, and wants a simple plan to increase their level of fitness significantly.

Time	Physical Activity Goals
Month 1	Begin P90X3 program.
Month 2	P90X3
Month 3	P90x3
Month 4	Begin T25 program.
Month 5	T25
Month 6	Favorite P90X3 or T25 workout 6 days per week.

REFERENCES

General Complaints

"Anaphylaxis—Overview." FamilyDoctor.org, April 2014. Accessed January 12, 2016.

Head

Clinch, C. Randall. "Evaluation of Acute Headaches in Adults." *American Family Physician* 63, no. 4 (February 2001): 685–693.

Eyes

"Eye Pain—Is It an Emergency?" All About Vision.com, June 2015. Accessed January 12, 2016.

Ears, Nose, and Throat

Fayad, J. N., and A. De La Cruz. "Etiologies and Treatment Options for Sudden Sensorineural Hearing Loss." *Hearing Review* 10, no. 13, (December 2003): 20–23.

Lieberthal, Allan S., Aaron E. Carroll, Tasnee Ganiats Chonmaitree, et al. "The Diagnosis and Management of Acute Otitis Media." *Pediatrics* 131, no. 3 (March 2013).

Back

"Low Back Pain Red Flags." *Family Practice Notebook.* fpnotebook. com, March 8, 2014. Accessed January 12, 2016.

Urinary System

"Hematuria." Cleveland Clinic Center for Continuing Education. clevelandclinicmeded.com, January 2009. Accessed January 12, 2016.

Neurology

"Spot a Stroke—Stroke Warning Signs and Symptoms." American Stroke Association. strokeassociation.org/STROKEORG/WarningSigns/Stroke. Accessed January 12, 2016.

"Altered Mental Status." medicinenet.com, December 17, 2015. Accessed January 12, 2016.

Organizing Your Medical Information

Cohen-Cole, Steven A. *The Medical Interview: The Three-Function Approach* (St Louis, MO: Mosby-Year Book, 1991), 67–77.

Miracles of Modern Medicine

"Mortality and Cause of Death, 1900 v. 2010," UNC Carolina Population Center—Carolina Demography, June 16, 2014. demography.cpc.unc.edu/2014/06/16/mortality-and-cause-of-death-1900-v-2010. Accessed January 14, 2016.

"Leading Causes of Death." Centers for Disease Control and Prevention—Fast Stats, September 30, 2013. cdc.gov/nchs/fastats/leading-causes-of-death.htm. Accessed January 14, 2016.

Ehreth, J. "The Global Value of Vaccination." *Vaccine* 21 (2003): 596–600.

"Adverse Effects of Vaccines Evidence and Causality." Institute of Medicine of the National Academies, August 2011. http://iom.nationalacademies.org/~/media/Files/Report%20Files/2011/Adverse-Effects-of-Vaccines-Evidence-and-Causality/Vaccine-report-brief-FINAL.pdf. Accessed January 14, 2016.

"Statins for Prevention of Cardiovascular Disease in Adults: Systematic Review for the U.S. Preventive Services Task Force." Agency for Healthcare Research and Quality U.S. Department of Health and Human Services, December 2015. file:///C:/Users/Demo. OxTab11241002/Downloads/statinsdraftes%20(1).pdf. Accessed January 14, 2016.

High Blood Pressure

James, Paul A., Suzanne Oparil, Barry L. Carter, et al. "2014 Evidence-Based Guideline for the Management of High Blood Pressure in Adults: Report from the Panel Members Appointed to the Eighth Joint National Committee (JNC 8)." *Journal of the American Medical Association* 311, no. 5 (2014): 507–520.

"2012 ACCF/AHA/ACP/AATS/PCNA/SCAI/STS Guideline for the Diagnosis and Management of Patients with Stable Ischemic Heart Disease." *Circulation* 125 (2012): e354–e471.

The *Be Healthy!* Workbook

On Being Healthy

Kochanek, Kenneth D., Sherry L. Murphy, and Jiaquan Xu. "Deaths: Final Data for 2011." *National Vital Statistics Report* 63, no. 3 (2015).

Losing Weight

Johnston, Bradley C., Steve Kanters, and Kristofer Bandayrel. "Comparison of Weight Loss among Named Diet Programs in Overweight and Obese Adults: A Meta-analysis." *JAMA* 312, no. 9 (2014): 923–933. doi:10.1001/jama.2014.10397.

"NWCR Facts." The National Weight Control Registry. nwcr.ws/Research. Accessed January 17, 2016.

Nutrition 101

"Mediterranean Diet 101." Oldways. oldwayspt.org. Accessed January 17, 2016.

"What Is Nutrient Density and Why Is It So Important?" *The World's Healthiest Foods.* Whfoods.org. http://www.whfoods.com/genpage. php?tname=george&dbid=81. Accessed January 17, 2016.

"Lose Weight Around the Clock." *The 8-Hour Diet.* 8hourdietbook. com. Accessed January 17, 2016.

Assignment: Controlling Eating Behavior

Reynolds, Gretchen. "A Twelve-Hour Window for a Healthy Weight." *New York Times,* January 15, 2015.

Assignment: Portion Control

"Serving Size Card." nhlbi.nih.gov/health/educational/wecan/downloads/ servingcard7.pdf, September 30, 2013. Accessed January 17, 2016.

"8 Tips for Controlling Portion Sizes: Use Portion Control Plates." *Health.* health.com/health/gallery/0,,20405321_7,00.html. Accessed January 17, 2016.

"Beauty." *ThePhilosophyofAndyWarhol.*http://thephilosophyofandywarhol. blogspot.com/2009/09/4-beauty.html.

Optimal Nutrition

"Mediterranean Diet 101." *Oldways.* oldwayspt.org. Accessed January 17, 2016.

Physical Activity

"How Much Physical Activity Do Adults Need?" Centers for Disease Control and Prevention: Division of Nutrition, Physical Activity, and

Obesity, June 4, 2015. http://www.cdc.gov/physicalactivity/basics/adults/index.htm. Accessed January 17, 2016.

"How Much Exercise Is Enough?" *Harvard Gazette,* November 6, 2012. news.harvard.edu/gazette. Accessed January 17, 2016.

"Exercise Intensity Matters More Than Duration in Keeping Weight Off: Study." *Huffpost Healthy Living.* huffingtonpost.com, September 4, 2013. Accessed January 17, 2016.

"Does Exercise Intensity Matter?" The Cooper Institute. cooperinstitute.org, July 18, 2011. Accessed January 17, 2016.

"10 Minute Workout: Short, Intense Workout to Get Fit." *Huffpost Healthy Living.* huffingtonpost.com, February 4, 2013. Accessed January 17, 2016.